SPIRITUALITY
IN THE 21ST CENTURY

FIFTH EDITION

Frank P. Daversa

Copyright © 2019 by Frank P. Daversa.

ISBN   Softcover   978-1-950580-02-6

All rights reserved. No part of this book may be reproduced or transmitted in any form or by any means, electronic or mechanical, including photocopying, recording, or by any information storage and retrieval system without express written permission from the author, except in the case of brief quotations embodied in critical reviews and certain other non-commercial uses permitted by copyright law.

Printed in the United States of America.

To order additional copies of this book, contact:
Bookwhip
1-855-339-3589
https://www.bookwhip.com

Contents

Introduction ix
Chapter 1 - Spiritual Growth: A Synopsis 1
Chapter 2 - In the Beginning 7
Chapter 3 - Karma and Paths 14
Chapter 4 - Spiritual Growth 18
Chapter 5 - Understanding Enlightenment 28
Chapter 6 - Achieving Enlightenment 32
Chapter 7 - Three Lessons 47
Chapter 8 - Wants vs. Needs 53
Chapter 9 - The Relative Value of Success 58
Chapter 10 - Love Relationship 65
Chapter 11 - Sins and Virtues,
 Religion and Death 75
Chapter 12 - Truth and Growth 92
Chapter 13 - Intolerance 98
Chapter 14 - Levels and Learning 104
Chapter 15 - Conclusion 115
Recommended Reading 118

*To all those who yearn for meaning
in their lives
and a vision with which to achieve it.*

Acknowledgments

I wish to thank the 50 or so people who read various stages of my original synopsis over the three-year period in which I developed it. The synopsis proved to be the springboard for this book, and the feedback I received from these individuals was instrumental in its evolution.

I am sincerely grateful to my sister, Geraldine Daversa, and my late cousin, Irene Benanti, for reading through my manuscript not once, but on two separate occasions. I needed a second and third set of eyes to tell me if I was on the right track, and they graciously provided their input, supplying valuable feedback that helped me make the manuscript the finished book it is today.

Portions excerpted from *BEYOND RELIGION: Ethics for a Whole World* by His Holiness the Dalai Lama. Copyright © 2011 by His Holiness the Dalai Lama. Reprinted by permission of Houghton Mifflin Harcourt Publishing Company. All rights reserved.

WHERE DO I BEGIN (From Paramount's Picture "Love Story"), Written by Francis Lai & Carl Sigman.
©1971 Sony/ATV Harmony (ASCAP), Music Sales Corp. (ASCAP).
All Rights by Sony/ATV Music Publishing LLC, 8 Music Sq. W., Nashville, TN. 37203.
All Rights Reserved. Used By Permission.

Introduction

*"It takes a person who is wide awake
to make his dream come true."*

—Roger Babson

Frank P. Daversa

Where do I begin, to tell the story of how great a love can be . . . is the opening refrain to a love song, the theme to the movie *Love Story* (1970). The song speaks of the difficulty the songwriter has in finding the words to express the extent of his emotion for the one he truly loves. I confess I am confronted with a similar dilemma, but one not limited to matters of the heart—as important as they may be. Rather, explaining spirituality challenges the very notion of who we are, where we have been, and where we are going together as a people, a society, and a species.

I will try to solve this dilemma using the concepts I present within this book. I hope my ideas ultimately enhance your understanding of spirituality, life, and the world as much as they have enhanced mine. Many people might feel these three concepts are part of some great mystery that cannot truly be solved; this need not be the case. Answers always exist—as long as you know where to find them. It is my intention to provide you with such answers and give you the insight and tools for finding your own.

Before I begin, let me state that this book is designed to provide hope and guidance for those starting out on their spiritual journeys, those not currently satisfied with the extent of their spiritual development and those wanting to otherwise enhance the spiritual part of their lives. **Please note that it is not intended to be an exhaustive discussion of the subject; instead,**

this book is meant to make you think, and to be a primer that starts you down the path toward spiritual self-discovery. In Particular, it focuses primarily on achieving the crown jewel of spirituality: spiritual enlightenment.

In an effort to appeal to as many different faiths as possible, I strive to be nondenominational in this book (aside from bringing up Jesus Christ). I was born a Roman Catholic, so my understanding of religion is based on the Cristian faith; my knowledge of other faiths consists largely of my reading as well as life experiences, which I draw upon wherever possible to make the subject matter easier to relate to. While certain religions refer to the Creator by different names, feel free to think of Him in turns of your own faith; many of the principles I describe here are applicable to a wide range of beliefs. I refer to Him here as God since that is how He is best known to me.

My book deals with spirituality, and spirituality is at the core of every religion. Many of the concepts I present tend to fall outside the tenets of most mainstream religions. Although I try not to adhere to any particular faith, you will find the book still shares beliefs in common with more than one of them.

As for my personal beliefs, I consider myself to be spiritual but not religious, and the book is essentially written from that perspective. This is not to say that one view is right and the other is wrong; all it means is that I believe the methods I present are better for many, if not most, people.

This book focuses mainly on growth—in particular, spiritual growth. As such, it covers many topics, from belief in God to spiritual paths, from truth to spiritual enlightenment. Unlike other more weighty texts of its kind, this book attempts to discuss these important topics in an easy-to-understand fashion. I hope you find I was successful in this regard.

As you read this book, I encourage you to apply my principles to your own goals. You may find that some of these principles are more challenging than others. Strive toward them gradually, but steadily. It will require commitment and time on your part in order to succeed. If pursued with diligence, these ideas should help you begin to experience the growth process, and thus acquire wisdom and inner peace when you're through. It's my earnest wish and intent that this book will answer more questions than it raises, but every reader will be different and perhaps have a different interpretation. It took a lifetime of experience and years of personal development and research for me to formulate these concepts, and even more to put them into words. They document my strongly held beliefs about spirituality, and I hope they possess significant meaning for you, too. Remember that we can't achieve all our goals overnight; they represent ongoing works in progress. Let the pursuit of them make as positive a difference in your life as it has in mine. Since these ideas are too important to keep all to myself, it's with great anticipation and utmost sincerity that I share them with you now.

Chapter 1
Spiritual Growth: A Synopsis

*"A man may die, nations may rise
and fall, but an idea lives on.
Ideas have endurance without death."*

—John F. Kennedy

Spirituality means different things to different people, but I define it as having a close and personal relationship with God and the universe. Enlightenment, on the other hand, represents a deep understanding of spirituality, ourselves, the needs of others, life, and nature.

I have a genuine interest in spirituality, and I try to embrace it in my personal life. Since 1997 I have been engaged in a spiritual journey that has inspired me to fully develop my faith in God. I originally conceived my thesis, in rudimentary form, almost three years prior to writing this book. After a good degree of soul searching, my initial quest for spiritual truth resulted in the passage which follows.

We Are Born with Default Paths
Based on my own experience and my observations of other people and different faiths, I sincerely believe that we all begin life with a default destiny, a spiritual path that God has chosen for us as only He sees fit. This path will guide us in a general direction, much like a leaf floating down a stream. Unlike the leaf, however, we possess the ability to think and the gift of free will, which enables us to change our default paths for better or worse during the course of our lifetimes, in turn creating new paths for ourselves.

Sometimes our default paths are especially good, but sometimes they're just mediocre or especially hard; for example, the families into which we're born could be nurturing or neglectful, loving or abusive. The best way to rise above our default paths is to grow spiritually. The more we grow, the greater our rewards, either in this life or in the life beyond.

God loves His children and wants us to grow closer to Him. A very effective way for us to grow is to become more aware of ourselves and the world around us. One person who greatly exemplified this idea was Dr. Martin Luther King, Jr. He was keenly aware of the needs of others in society, and he fought for those needs his whole life. Given his faith in God and his message of peace and love, Dr. King was most certainly rewarded with a special place in the afterlife.

There are many problems in the world today. Naturally, the most effective means of eradicating a problem is to eliminate its cause or source. For example, illegal drugs are a dilemma in our society; the best approach for solving this problem is to stop the demand for drugs through education and interdiction. On a personal level, many problems arise because people have dysfunctions in their lives, often resulting in a void—something is missing. One important factor commonly missing in our society today is a cohesive family structure. Problem families create voids in both adults' and children's lives, in turn affecting children developmentally. These developmental difficulties often multiply into adulthood.

Five Fundamental Principles of Spiritual Enlightenment

While family counseling begins to correct the problem, an excellent way to fill such a void is through *spiritual enlightenment*. Spiritual enlightenment helps people to build moral character and become more complete individuals, which leads to better relationships, stronger families, and more fulfilling lives. There is more than one path toward enlightenment, but a very effective way is to become spiritually one with God, ourselves, and the world around us through love and devotion for Him. Oneness, a union of mind, body, and spirit into a greater celestial whole, is a unique and unparalleled experience. To achieve both, thoughtfully practice these five principles:

1. Accept God into your life and Jesus Christ as your savior;
2. Complete your formal education;
3. Learn more about yourself, your health and your mental well-being;
4. Learn more about the needs of others;

5. Learn more about the natural environment in which we live.

This kind of understanding will help us attain a greater degree of wisdom and inner peace, giving us guidance to make responsible choices in life. This is especially true for young children, since they generally embrace faith and spirituality naturally. Once we fill the void in this manner, the problem will most likely be solved.

Rising Above Our Default Paths

There exists an absolute truth in life, and only God knows it. The more we grow spiritually, the more we begin to comprehend that truth. Earth is merely a learning ground for humanity to evolve spiritually before moving on to the afterlife. As with any form of education, learning involves lessons. We can either learn our spiritual lessons proactively or passively—either way, God will see to it that those lessons will be learned. If together we learn proactively, we will rise above our default spiritual paths and have the chance to lead happy, fulfilling lives. If we learn passively, we rely instead on our default paths, and we will then be destined to either repeat the lessons or learn them the hard way.

World Wars I and II are two 20th-century examples of how we learned lessons the hard way. In both wars, world powers didn't heed the threats of tyranny, appeasement, and imperialism far enough in advance, so many nations had to pay a heavy price to defeat these threats after the fact. An example of learning proactively is the 1991 Persian Gulf War, in which the global community mobilized its military forces against a tyrant before it was too late. The result was a war that lasted only a few months with far fewer casualties than other wars.

Three very important spiritual challenges to overcome in this century are global warming, overpopulation, and environmental degradation. Unless we reduce the buildup of greenhouse gases in the atmosphere and undo the damage we have done to the environment, the world will become a fairly inhospitable place and millions of people will suffer needlessly as a result. Together, we can prevail over these challenges if we act now rather than later.

This synopsis summarizes most of the major concepts I believe about spirituality. It is safe to say that if you like what you have read, then you will like what follows. The inverse is also true. The five principles are provided for your personal enlightenment. If followed as intended, they should guide you toward new spiritual heights. The remainder of this book is dedicated to explaining these and other concepts in greater detail. I hope it is as rewarding for you to read as it was for me to write. So let the journey begin . . .

Chapter 2
In the Beginning . . .

"Develop a passion for learning. If you do, you will never cease to grow."

—Anthony J. D'Angelo

What makes people who they are? Genetic and environmental influences shape us from the day we are born, factors over which we have limited control until we reach puberty. But one other factor is sometimes overlooked in secular society: our souls.

Our souls contribute toward shaping the people we are, thus influencing our paths in life, namely the default spiritual path God assigned each of us at birth. Sometimes this default path is especially beneficial; other times it's just mediocre; sometimes it's plain bad. Our spiritual goals in life should be to make the most of our paths if they are good ones and to strive to rise above them and define new ones if they are not.

My Obstacles to Spiritual Living
Over time, my default path has become apparent to me: I realized that I have been different emotionally from others since the day I was born. Emotions make up such a large part of our personalities, it's no wonder being challenged in this way caused me to stand out from most people.

My family was dysfunctional in many ways, which undoubtedly shaped me at an early age. To start with, everything I know emotionally I had to learn on my own—I received little guidance from them. I had to pull myself up by my own bootstraps in this regard. My family's emotional behavior tended to be erratic, which led me to respond in the same way, something which I had to overcome in later years. At times, their behavior was like a roller coaster, which made leading a normal life a real challenge. Second, there was often little patience between family members, frequently resulting in short tempers and semi-intolerant behavior. Third, they typically failed to validate each other's feelings, leading to a sense of insecurity, at least on my part.

Grade school was especially difficult. My family lived at the edge of our school district, far from most kids who went to my school, which largely left me underdeveloped socially as a child. Outside of a couple of close friends, I was unsuccessful at socializing with most children. This obstacle was endlessly frustrating, since I was perpetually cast as the outlier. Eventually, I began longing for any and all information that could help explain why I was different.

For whatever reason, God had decided that I would not begin to blossom until I reached adulthood. It wasn't until I reached college age that I began to understand the problem: While I possessed the tools to develop intellectually, I was underdeveloped emotionally. Being deprived of emotional guidance while growing up, I tended to be needy throughout my youth. I was more successful socially in college—I belonged to a group of about eight friends for most of my time there, and I am friends with some even to this day. Despite that, I still needed assistance with life's issues. Eventually, I began seeing a therapist, which proved to be enormously helpful. Of course, she couldn't undo a lifetime of problems in just one college semester, but my sessions with her gave me the tools I needed for starting down the path of self-realization. You can't solve a problem until you first understand it, which is why "Learn more about yourself, your health and your mental well-being" is one of my five principles of spiritual enlightenment.

A couple of years later, I came across a book that further changed my life forever: *A Guide to Rational Living,* by Albert Ellis, Ph.D., and Robert A. Harper, Ph.D. It helped me understand the relationship between my thoughts, emotions, and behaviors in a way I had never known before, a way that helped me understand my specific problems and how to resolve them. At last, I had tools I could use to rise above my limitations!

I was finally able to exercise free will to advance beyond my default path and define a new path for myself, one that was much more fulfilling than the original one. I realized that although my default path was preordained, my new path was not. I could make it whatever I wanted it to be, preferably one more rewarding in nature.

Trying to do some good

One prime example of an adverse default path occurred with my brother's eldest son. He had been having trouble with his grades in high school, so my brother and I decided to relocate him to Houston to live and go to school there. Up until 1992, my brother and his family lived in New York and I, of course, lived in Houston. We scheduled visits for him to the city a few times in the past, hence he was familiar with the place. So my 16-year-old nephew moved in with me in the summer of 1991. My brother and I arranged it so that I would be his legal guardian. Things went as well as could be expected at first.

Then transference began to set in. The problems he had at home with his parents soon began to surface. Being the only authority figure, I bore the brunt of his teenage wrath and rebellion. Getting him to go to bed on time was impossible and getting him up for school was nearly as difficult. His room looked like a neutron bomb hit it: the place was a wreck, but the walls were still standing. You see, one of the main problems with my nephew was his mind was empty of knowledge. He was a classic example of the consequences of having a void in one's life. He was also immature for his age. I hold his parents foremost responsible for these shortcomings. The key word describing the cause of my nephew's behavior up to this point is *neglect*.

By the end of the second quarter in school, I had gone about as far as I could go with him. I desperately needed professional help. In January of 1992, I admitted him, with his consent, into a psychiatric hospital south of where we lived. Finally, there were professionals to share the responsibility of helping him grow up. He began going to school at the hospital. I would visit him there a couple of times a week, and after a while he was granted weekend passes to spend at home.

Months passed without much incident, except for the death of his maternal grandmother. The two were very close, and my nephew, of course, wanted to attend her funeral. She lived in New York, so I arranged his flight up there. Naturally, this would mean he would take time off from the hospital. There was a concern he would not return to it upon coming back, but fortunately he did. Outside of this, things proceeded as smoothly as could be expected until my brother lost his job and announced he was taking the opportunity to relocate to Houston, also. So my brother and his family moved there late in the summer of 1992.

My nephew's psychiatrist saw this as an opportunity to unload a problem child and announced he was being released from the hospital. I saw red. The work the hospital was doing with him was not nearly as finished as it needed to be. His parents welcomed the change. They had priority over me; there was nothing I could do.

He was released in the fall of 1992 during his senior year of high school. Considering the problems he had with his family, we all agreed he would live with me for his 12th year of schooling. Unfortunately, my nephew decided not to complete school at that time. So he lived with me for a year until fall 1993 when he finally got the gumption to go back to school. The hospital did some good in that he attended of his own volition. He managed to complete his final year with passing grades which was an accomplishment. At this point, there was little need for him to stay with me, so he moved back in with his parents and they resumed being a content but dysfunctional family.

I wish I could say his stay with me was a success, but there was so much more work that needed to be done with him. It was successful in one regard though: he graduated high school. And I'd like to think his head was a little less empty. You see, every shortcoming inherent in my family was realized in my nephew. For whatever reason, God saw fit that this would be his default path in life. I tried to change the course of history and in a small but essential way I did. I have yet to have any children, but I certainly got a taste of raising a child after all of this. Needless to say, my personal life was at a standstill while all this happened. Spiritual work is seldom easy (even though my primary goal was to get him through school).

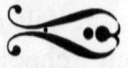

Chapter 3
Karma and Paths

"Each man is the architect of his own fate."

—Appius Claudius

As previously stated, default paths are spiritual paths God assigns to us at birth. The basic premise of karma is the belief that a person's actions during his or her lifetime affect how he or she will be reincarnated into the next life. It is practiced by Hindus, Buddhists, Sikhs, and Jains, to name a few.

According to the Hindu religion, karma is the cycle of cause and effect that governs all life, brought on by our actions and deeds. To cite Paramhans Swami Maheshwarananda, "Everything we have ever thought, spoken, done, or caused is karma, as is also that which we think, speak, or do this very moment."

In Buddhist theory, the nature of our deeds, for better or worse, is not the only factor that affects our karma. Our individual natures, as well as the circumstances surrounding our deeds, also determine our path in the next life. For example, although the taking of a life is a mortal sin that might condemn a person in the next lifetime, if the person taking the life is a spiritual person who did so in self-defense, there might not be a negative karmic effect.

One difference between karma and spiritual paths is that karma is inherited from a previous life that can't be altered, whereas default paths are assigned by God at birth and can be altered by free will. Another difference is that karma is largely represented by a two-sided cause-and-effect scale: The greater the number of good deeds you perform on one side, the greater the number of rewards you receive on the other (likewise for bad deeds). In other words, what goes around comes around. It's possible for someone to perform good deeds with good intentions and receive rewards, but not grow all that much as a person. For instance, you could donate regularly to charity, but only for the tax deduction, feeling little or no empathy for the people to whom you're donating. In this case, although you might achieve good karma, you're not raising your consciousness and will remain somewhat stunted in your personal and/or spiritual development.

Spiritual Growth
Spiritual paths revolve around growth—a deed may not necessarily result in a karmic reward, but rather in spiritual growth, which is its own reward. In other words, good things usually happen from good deeds. For instance, the item you donate to the Salvation Army could be rejected because they already have too many of the same thing, so you wouldn't get the tax deduction or be able to perform the good deed you'd intended. However, even though you didn't receive a reward, your intentions were good, so you would experience some personal growth.

The more we grow, the more assured we become of receiving positive outcomes for our efforts. The further we develop spiritually, the more fulfilling and enriched our lives will be.

I contend it's possible that God directs our spirits to accomplish goals in other lifetimes. Although Eastern religions claim our future lives are dictated by the laws of karma, I believe such transformations are dictated by God Himself. One potential purpose of divine interventions like these might be to give us the opportunity to achieve a greater good in our new lives or to finish learning something we didn't sufficiently learn in our previous ones. On the other hand, you may have lived a full life with little unfinished business upon passing and hence don't need to be reincarnated, but I believe it is possible at least for some.

Upon being reborn, God assigns us new default spiritual paths which may or may not be favorable. We can still advance beyond such paths and improve upon them over the course of our inherited lifetimes. When we finally achieve a high state of consciousness, we cease to be reborn and move on to a more enlightened spiritual level in the afterlife. Whether we are reincarnated or born anew, we can make the most of our lives by defining better paths for ourselves.

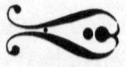

Chapter 4
Spiritual Growth

"To be what we are, and to become what we are capable of becoming, is the only end of life."

—Robert Louis Stevenson

"Life isn't about finding yourself. Life is about creating yourself."

—George Bernard Shaw

People born onto difficult spiritual paths may have to endure considerable hardship in order to rise above their challenges—such is God's will. Some people believe adversity is natural, that we must suffer and sacrifice in order to purge our souls of sin so that we can grow spiritually and achieve a state of enlightenment. But although hardship may present sufficient conditions for growth, it's not the only way to learn. Otherwise, people born onto easier spiritual paths would hardly ever reach enlightenment!

A Thoughtful Approach to Spirituality
Eliminating all forms of discomfort is neither possible nor beneficial—challenge is good for the soul—but we can also learn without suffering. For instance, we can pursue a good education and seek out good role models from which to learn. If you yearn for wisdom as much as I do, you will benefit from insights obtained in a more formal manner. I believe that the more you expose your mind to new ideas, the more you will want to explore them and grow. Finding the right path isn't necessarily easy, but it need not seem impossible, either. My goal is to help get as many people as possible started on a new, real path toward spiritual enlightenment, not make them hesitant to even try. Many people living in poverty are confronted with so many obstacles

that they feel compelled to give up right from the start.

Unless we were fortunate enough to be born onto a very favorable path, we'll encounter challenges to overcome and lessons to learn along the way. If we meet these challenges, we'll have the opportunity to define new paths for ourselves; if not, then we'll remain stagnant and at the mercy of our default spiritual paths, whatever they happen to be.

Like many people, I have suffered to achieve what I have learned—more than some, but less than others. I didn't have someone to earnestly guide me toward a path of enlightenment. Although I received valuable advice along the way with regard to specific life issues, I didn't have anyone explain for me the "big picture." I was a lost soul looking for guidance. I had to attain what I understand mostly through sheer trial and error. It was only when I reached a moderate level of enlightenment that I began to look back and realize there must be a better way to advance up the spiritual ladder.

Growth Is God's Plan for Us

Our purpose in life is to grow, spiritually and otherwise (such as careers and relationships). The journey toward spiritual enlightenment begins with empowerment, which in turn begins with sound ideas. Nothing is more powerful than a good idea—ideas have brought down ruthless dictatorships and inspired us to land on the moon. The more we expose our minds to new ideas, the more inclined we will be to explore these ideas and grow from them.

Look at what happened during the Dark Ages—learning and growth came to a virtual standstill on an individual and a societal level. Very little progressed for hundreds of years. Civilization and societies broke down and became fractured following the decline of the Roman Empire. People became preoccupied with survival and just living day to day. Contrast that period with the Renaissance—an explosion of new ideas resulted in growth in most areas of civilization. It developed as a result of a resurgence in such fields as literature, philosophy, art, music, politics, science, religion, and other intellectual pursuits. Today, people with new, innovative ideas are in demand in every sector of society. Imagine accomplishing such growth on a personal level—our lives could be so much richer.

Frank P. Daversa

A Presidential Example
No one better exemplifies the pattern of personal growth than President Ronald Reagan, who had to overcome several key hurdles which ultimately enabled him to become president. After becoming class president at Eureka College in his senior year, he was hired as a sportscaster in Davenport, Iowa, followed by a position as sports announcer for the Chicago Cubs. In 1937, while traveling with the team to Southern California, he took a screen test that led to a seven-year contract with Warner Brothers studios, which in turn led to success as a B-movie actor. He largely remained that way until 1941, when he was first elected to the board of directors of the Screen Actors Guild. In 1947 he was officially elected as president of the Guild and was subsequently renominated for seven additional one-year terms.

Reagan's first big political breakthrough began in 1966 when he was elected governor of California for two terms. In 1968 and 1976, he tested the presidential waters, vying for the Republican nomination; he lost both times. Many people in his position might have simply given up, but he persisted, and in 1980 he officially became the 40th president of the United States, an office in which he served for two terms as you well know.

As you can see, Reagan faced challenges in each stage of his career. Because he worked to overcome them, he eventually became president;

if he had not, he would have remained nothing more than a B-movie actor.

Reagan's skill set naturally prepared him for high office. If you were to "connect the dots" that make up his spiritual path, they naturally point toward a presidency. On the other hand, although I could have run for a low-level political office if I really wanted to (which I did *not*), there was nothing in my initial skill set to prepare me for such a path. Because of the direction my default spiritual path has taken me, I would have had to overcome enormous obstacles to achieve any kind of political success. Instead, I pursued my own spiritual path, building on the skills I possessed.

Personal Challenges

As an inherent part of my default path, each challenge represented a lesson in life. If I learned the lesson, I would advance to the next spiritual level available to me on Earth. If not, I was destined to either repeat the lesson or remain mired in the state of relative dysfunction in which I'd found myself. Of course, I acquired knowledge only in hindsight, but each time I did so, I was able to take the knowledge and apply it to another challenge down my path.

When I was 23 years old, I had no business skills to speak of. I had almost four years of college behind me and no degree to show for it. I was behind my age emotionally. I was going nowhere fast. Instead of settling on that path, I enrolled in a local community college at the advice of a friend and earned a degree in computer programming. By the time I graduated with honors in the fall of 1981, I already had my first job in the field.

I worked full time for a couple of years afterward, until I decided to return to school part time to complete my four-year college degree. Working and going to school was indeed tough, but by spring 1986, I had completed my bachelor's degree in computer science with a 3.96 GPA. In facing the challenge of what to do with the rest of my life, I created a new career for myself with real growth potential. I credit God and His divine guidance with steering me down this beneficial path to begin with.

As an adult, I always had an interest in communicating my thoughts through writing. The advent of email solidified that desire. As a result, the next professional challenge I faced was deciding in 2007 to become a writer. I had an idea for a book, and I made it happen. Here too, I took a chance and it paid off. If you had told me back in 1980, when I started on my first career path, that I would become a writer, I would have thought you were nuts! But looking back, much about my past has led me to this point in life. For example, I formulated what amounted to the introduction of this book as far back as the year

2000 for a work on spirituality and science that was never realized.

Fast-forward to the present. Driving home one evening, I was listening to a disc jockey who gives personal advice on the air. She was talking about what lies ahead for us, and then she said something that both astounded and offended me: We have no control over our futures. She said we can't even control a sneeze, let alone our own destinies, and all we can do is just worry about the present.

I was stunned. Countless people listen to this woman for advice, and she turns around and tells them they can't control their own destinies? While there's something to be said for living in the moment, you'd better plan for the future, too, which certainly means that you can shape your own destiny. I spent 30 years of my life creating two different career paths for myself, and she tells me it can't be done? A sneeze might be involuntary, but our futures are not. We can always create new paths for ourselves, as long as we have the determination. If I could do it, then so could you.

You Define the Meaning of Your Life
Only you can determine the meaning of your life. Most people do so in terms of their careers or vocations, so choose a path that interests you deeply, as it will ultimately guide you. We can't

find meaning in an experiential vacuum, which is why education is so important. Education broadens our minds, teaches us to think critically, and makes us more worldly. Bear in mind that regardless of the career path we choose for ourselves, we still may not surpass our default paths unless we grow spiritually. We can be almost anything we want to be—we just have to weigh the pros and cons of our choices. This is not to say that we must face these challenges all on our own; praying for guidance is a natural and important means by which to communicate with God. We may not get a response every time, but our concerns will always be heard.

As we follow our spiritual paths, if we learn our lessons well, we'll earn the right to define better paths for ourselves. Keep in mind that we can't always tell in advance what direction our path is going to take—the important thing is to keep moving in a positive direction regardless of where we think we might be headed.

There is no reward for complacency. It's very important to responsibly choose a path and then pursue it. You'll soon discover whether it's the right one for you; if not, take a few steps back and select another one. The key is to keep trying—God rewards effort. Many times the reward will come in this life; other times, in the life beyond. Either way, the reward will be realized. More often than not, we will find there really is a pot of gold at the end of the rainbow, so long as we choose our paths wisely.

Spiritual growth encompasses everything around us. It represents a holistic and heightened understanding of God, ourselves, the people surrounding us, and our environment—the universe as a whole. This kind of awareness helps us grow more completely as individuals. No one better exemplified this level of development than Dr. Martin Luther King, Jr. His many marches, protests, and speeches demonstrate that he was keenly aware of the needs of others in society, something for which he fought his whole life. He most certainly was rewarded a special place in the afterlife.

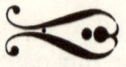

Chapter 5
Understanding Enlightenment

"A good head and a good heart are always a formidable combination."

—Nelson Mandela

War, terrorism, hunger, and human rights abuses are just a few of the problems our world faces today. The most effective means of eradicating a problem is to eliminate its cause. For example, a major cause of hunger is poverty. Eliminate poverty, and you will likely eliminate hunger in much of the world. Illegal drugs are also a dilemma in society; the best way to resolve that problem is to stop the demand for drugs through education and interdiction. On a personal level, many problems arise because people have dysfunctions in their lives, often because something is missing. For example, millions of people find it impossible to rise out of poverty because they lack a formal education. Educate poor people and you will significantly reduce poverty.

Family Is the Foundation
One important factor often missing in our society today is a cohesive family structure. Many families experience marital problems, destructive sibling rivalries, and a lack of respect for family members in general. Because something is missing, one can say there is a *void* in their lives. Problem families create voids in children's lives, in turn affecting them developmentally. For example, children need to develop in a loving home, and when marital problems exist, their fragile self-esteems can suffer. Difficulties

such as these often multiply into adulthood. Low self-esteem early on can lead to depression later in life. Although family counseling can put families on the road toward resolving their problems, spiritual enlightenment can enhance the process significantly. Spiritual enlightenment builds moral character and enables people to feel complete, which leads to better relationships, stronger families, and more fulfilling lives. It helps you to become more knowledgeable and worldly, thus giving you the tools to make better decisions in life. It helps you to become more compassionate, thus improving your ability to participate in relationships and interact with your fellow human beings. Knowing that God believes in you as much as you believe in Him gives you strength to face life's challenges.

Family counseling can be an important resource, as mentioned above. A counselor can help resolve some of the personal and relationship issues underlying a family's problems, but a real, long-term solution must go beyond simple family counseling to include the concept of spiritual enlightenment.

Enlightenment Builds Character
Building moral character enables us to become more complete as people, which leads to better relationships, stronger families, and more fulfilling lives. Enlightenment helps us develop a greater understanding of God and the issues involved in life and society. The more aware and worldly we are, the better we will be able to face the challenges that impact our lives.

Enlightenment can, subsequently, help us reach a state of oneness, which occurs when we develop a deep understanding of, or connectedness to, someone so fully that we are not only conscious of the person's presence, but we can also sense what he or she is thinking and feeling. We operate on the same wavelength, existing in complete harmony with the other person and/or our surroundings. For example, nature is a very spiritual realm, especially in its pristine state. When I experience a lush green meadow, not only do I *see* the flowers, grass, and trees, I *feel* them as well. I am completely in touch with the grandeur they represent. One way to achieve this state is to become one with ourselves, one with the world around us, and one with God through love and devotion for Him. Since spirituality facilitates oneness, such a state of being requires that we get in touch with our spirituality. Oneness is a unique experience, unequaled by others.

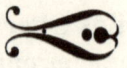

Chapter 6
Achieving Enlightenment

"Growth itself contains the [seed] of happiness."

—Pearl S. Buck

There is more than one way to achieve enlightenment—every religion has its own method for developing spiritually—but in order to achieve spiritual enlightenment, I contend we need to follow five timeless, fundamental principles.

Principle #1—Accept God into Your Life and Jesus Christ as Your Savior

God is the Supreme Being and Creator of all things on Earth and in the universe; His powers are infinite. As such, He can have an enormous impact on our lives. Simply put, we have to believe in God in order to grow spiritually; everything revolves around Him. Not enough can be said about Him. We must trust in Him. We must respect His awesome knowledge and strength, while fearing Him at the same time. We must never take Him for granted; instead, it is vital that we cherish His love. He is perfection. He is the ultimate arbiter of right and wrong. He passes final judgment on our souls when we advance into the afterlife. He is both absolute love and punishment. He only administers punishment when He has to; otherwise, He is unconditional and universal love. When we embrace God, He embraces us in His own way. He loves us deeply and wants us to grow closer to Him, but in order to truly grow closer, we must first grow spiritually. He has an elaborate plan to make that happen. It is important we learn from it sooner rather than later.

Also vital to spiritual growth is accepting Jesus Christ as our savior. Jesus Christ is God's only begotten son, and He sacrificed His life on the cross to bring salvation to humankind. Jesus brings us unconditional love and forgiveness for our sins. If we understand and share in the love He has for humanity, we will be a big step closer to enlightenment. Love for Jesus brings hope for a more spiritual and meaningful life.

I know firsthand what it means to be both a believer and a nonbeliever. Even though I grew up Catholic, I gradually became disenchanted with the church during my adolescence, and when I finally reached adulthood, I became an agnostic. I questioned whether there really was a God. During that time, I had minimal spiritual development. I remained that way for 20 years, until 1997, when I developed a recurring illness that changed my life forever.

I was diagnosed with schizoaffective disorder. My illness is characterized by psychotic episodes in which my thoughts suddenly become distorted and my emotions become withdrawn; it basically takes control of my life, putting me under a great deal of stress. During these episodes, it's a struggle just to think clearly. Everyday things no longer matter; all I want is to simply survive. The only things I can reliably focus on are my psychological problems. There is nothing anyone can do to help; I have to get through it on my own. Minutes feel like hours, and hours feel like days. Each time hopelessness would take over, I would say to myself, "Is this all there is to life?"

It was in my darkest hour that I realized that there was a void in my life—something was missing, something big. The further I looked within my soul, the more I realized it was my spiritual life that was lacking. At that point, I officially accepted God in my life once again. Suddenly, life no longer seemed hopeless. There was a master plan to everything in the universe, and in some way I was a part of it. I realized that upon becoming an agnostic, I had essentially fallen out of sync with the universe.

My illness was God's way of bringing me back into spiritual alignment. The years from 1998 through 2006 were especially traumatic. While I am enormously relieved those bad experiences are now behind me and I would never want to relive them again, I will say the hardships I endured made me emotionally stronger and more self-reliant in the end. My illness also served to restore my faith. While I still don't consider myself religious, I do regard myself as spiritual and maintain a strong belief in God, Jesus Christ, and the afterlife. The more I grew spiritually, the more my love for God grew and the more I appreciated the role He plays in my life. For me, growing closer to God and Jesus means following the tenets described in this book.

Frank P. Daversa

Principle #2—Complete Your Formal Education

It is difficult to approach enlightenment without first acquiring a basic understanding of how the world works, and the best way to do that is to educate yourself. Though I emphasize the value of a high school education, many of the concepts found in this book can be introduced to children in a scaled-down version while they're still young. This will help give them a head start in life before they take on more challenging topics as adults. This should be fairly easy to do: because of their innocence, young children generally embrace faith and spirituality naturally.

In the United States, it is both a privilege and a right to be educated. Many societies in the world deprive their citizens of a basic education. In places like these, women are denied such rights because of political or religious fundamentalism and are forced to either work in low-income jobs or dedicate their lives exclusively to raising a family. Children are made to work in factories or on farms for little or no wages. Neither of them have any chance of bettering themselves; they're faced with a lifetime of unskilled labor. Talk about being born into a poor default path . . .

So take advantage of an education if you have access to one. You will gain much-needed knowledge and the skills to think critically. This book is designed to give you a well-rounded understanding of spirituality, so it is only natural that you come similarly prepared.

Principle #3—Learn More About Yourself, Your Health & Your Mental Well-Being

Better understanding of ourselves and our bodies' needs is essential to understanding how to nurture our physical and spiritual beings. We can't effectively help ourselves grow unless we also take proper care of our overall health and nutritional needs. God gave us these bodies to use in this life, so make the most of them. Eat foods high in protein and low in saturated fat and cholesterol, maintain a normal body weight for your height, don't smoke, drink alcohol in moderation, and exercise regularly. Be of sound mind and body, and you'll have a more holistic life experience.

Self-discovery and self-realization are vital to getting further in touch with ourselves and achieving oneness. We are ultimately responsible for our own thoughts and behaviors. Most people take their thoughts and feelings for granted, but family, biological and environmental factors contribute to their creation. This is not to say we have to engage in the growth process all on our own; there are supportive tools we can use to accomplish this goal.

To become fully enlightened, we need to let go of our negative thoughts and emotions, ridding ourselves of them so that we can think clearly. One tool that worked very well for me is Ellis and Harper's *A Guide to Rational Living*, which discusses a concept known as REBT—Rational Emotive Behavioral Therapy. The book helps us to better understand the relationship between our thoughts, emotions, and behaviors and to determine how to make them function effectively.

The key to personal growth is training our minds; the more training we do, the happier and more at ease we'll be with ourselves. Both positive and negative thoughts arise from our perception of our experiences, depending on how disciplined we are. It's important to keep working at the growth process until we succeed. As His Holiness the Dalai Lama contends in his book *In My Own Words: An Introduction to My Teachings and Philosophy,* from this perspective, negative thoughts become weak and vulnerable. As soon as we see them for what they are and develop the sense to know better, we can effectively erase them, and once we eliminate negative thoughts within our minds, they can't return unless we let them. They can't reappear somewhere else and reinforce themselves like a conventional enemy could, so they can't return to harm us. To be ultimately successful, though, we must want to change for the better. To do so, we must visualize a life full of constructive ideas and largely free of negative ones. Once we make up our minds, we can think clearly.

Reading *A Guide to Rational Living* enabled me to eliminate my self-defeating behaviors and enhance my sense of self-awareness, a quality vital to personal growth. The book questioned some of my existing beliefs, teaching me that in order to be truly successful, I had to put aside my ego. I also learned how to deal better with adversity. Now when something negative happens, I try to remember that my resulting feelings won't last forever. In the end, I grew as a person and in my understanding of myself.

Principle #4—Learn More About the Needs of Others

The more we understand about ourselves, the more we'll understand how others behave, since we share needs in common with them. Only after accomplishing both will we truly be able to connect spiritually with another person. Compassion goes hand in hand with the Golden Rule. Implicit in that is having feelings for others as we encounter them. God wants us to have compassion and respect for our fellow human beings, especially those who are suffering greatly, such as the millions of people living in poverty, suffering from hunger, or experiencing human rights abuses. People have the same basic needs: food, shelter, happiness, companionship, etc.

Poor people use whatever means are available to them in order to fulfill their needs. Their default spiritual paths have forced them to focus primarily on their fundamental requirements rather than their material desires. I believe there is a lesson to be learned in that for all of us.

We must bear in mind two simple truths: just as we have instinctive and legitimate desires to be happy and avoid suffering, so do all other people; and just as we have the right to fulfill these innate aspirations, so do they. It is likely that the more we live by these truths, the more we will want to care for the happiness of others; hence the greater our sense of well-being will become. Compassion dictates that we assist those in need wherever possible.

Helping our fellow humans places us on a path toward self-realization. However, to be truly altruistic, we must first put our lives in perspective. His Holiness the Dalai Lama sums it up appropriately by saying that as important a person as one might be, the simple truth is that the happiness of many people is more important than the happiness of one individual. With this humble view in mind, it's possible to cultivate a sense of compassion, love, and respect for others. We really can make the world a better place if we all work together.

A good place to begin improving the world would be raising the standard of living for developing countries. On a broad scale, the business community needs to contribute toward solving problems inherent to developing nations. It's incumbent upon developed nations to use their abundant resources to help citizens of developing countries improve their lives through such areas as better manufacturing techniques, educational systems, and health care. However, it is important to remember that one cannot improve economic opportunity without effecting social change as well.

As His Holiness the Dalai Lama states in his book *In My Own Words: An Introduction to My Teachings and Philosophy*:

> Tremendous effort will be required to bring compassion into the realm of international business. Economic inequality, especially that between developed and developing nations, remains the greatest source of suffering on this planet. Even though [money will be lost] in the short term, large multinational corporations must curtail their exploitation of poor nations. Tapping the few precious resources such countries possess simply to fuel consumption in the developed world is disastrous; if it continues unchecked, eventually we shall all suffer. Strengthening weak, undiversified economies is a far wiser policy for promoting both political and economic stability. As idealistic as it may sound, altruism, not just competition and the desire for wealth, should be a driving force in business.

Frank P. Daversa

There will always be problems in the world as long as there exists a great divide between the haves and have-nots. Desperate people tend to resort to desperate measures to satisfy their needs. It is inherently unethical for certain people to fulfill their material desires at the expense of others' fundamental necessities. Consider the wealthiest among us—a study by Oxfam found that the richest 1% of the world's population controls nearly 50% of global wealth. In the United States, the Congressional Budget Office reports between 1979 and 2007 incomes of the top 1% of the population grew by an average of 275% while the lower 90% lagged far behind. Furthermore, the 400 richest Americans have more wealth than the bottom 150 million combined, according to Berkeley Professor and former Labor Secretary Robert Reich. These numbers are staggering, and they underscore the income inequality that exists in this country alone. They beg the question, how much wealth is enough?

If it is measured as a percentage of U.S. Gross Domestic Product, then it is undoubtedly too much. Even Pope Francis denounced income inequality in his 2013 Evangelii Gaudium. Wealth is too concentrated at the top and those at the bottom are not sharing in that success. The point here is not that the rich should randomly give away their wealth to the poor, but at least invest their good fortune in those who support their bottom line. An excellent place to start would be raising the minimum wage so full-time workers can live above the poverty line. A company's employees work hard to promote its financial success; why not return the favor by compassionately increasing their salaries to a living wage? Maybe then they would not have to depend so much here in the U.S. on government assistance such as Medicaid, CHIP (Children's Health Insurance Program), and SNAP (Supplemental Nutrition Assistance Program).

As we expand our understanding of people in need, hopefully our desire to help them will grow in kind, and we'll search for ways to become involved. A great place to begin is through CARE (care.org), one of the world's largest private international humanitarian organizations fighting global poverty and social injustice. The nation's premier emergency response organization, the American Red Cross (redcross.org) provides vital humanitarian assistance to victims of war and natural disasters (the international partner of the Red Cross is the International Committee of the Red Cross, or icrc.org). Amnesty International (amnestyusa.org) is the world's largest grassroots human rights organization. They envision a world in which every person enjoys all of the human rights enumerated in the Universal Declaration of Human Rights (UDHR) and other internationally recognized human rights standards.

I encourage everyone to donate to one of these reputable organizations or a related charity of your choice. As long as there are people in this world, we will all have to work together to make it a better place in which to live and grow. Most charities have the know-how to do just that, so they are a good place to start. Remembering that no man is an island represents the first step toward living with and helping others.

Principle #5—Learn More About the Natural Environment in Which We Live

Nature is very spiritual—it represents beauty and sustenance. God designed nature to be inherently beautiful for our benefit so that we would learn to appreciate and respect it. Sustenance represents survival. Hence becoming one with nature is among the most spiritual experiences we can possibly undertake. Because nature and the environment are deeply interconnected, what we do to the environment will also have spiritual repercussions.

As a species, we are as dependent upon the environment as the earth is dependent on the sun. To ignore or disregard this fact is to put our heads firmly in the sand. The more we understand the environment, the more we can do to improve it—and it's important to our spiritual paths that we do both.

God gave us this planet as a paradise to use as He envisioned. He has allowed us a wide degree of latitude to do with it as we like, but there are limits to how far we can go before we destroy the world or make it largely uninhabitable. Global warming is a classic example—we need to reduce greenhouse gas emissions—primarily carbon dioxide—on a global scale, or the consequences will be dire: Temperatures will rise, polar ice caps will melt, sea levels will rise, and climates will drastically change. This isn't news—it's already begun. God is sending us a warning with the severe, unseasonal and unusual storms, tornadoes, and other natural disasters we have been experiencing as of late, but we are not adequately heeding His message. If we don't act now, the time will come when we will have to answer directly to Him for our inactions.

Although much of what needs to be done has to be handled at the national and global level, the average person can still contribute to the solution. For instance, planting trees will help absorb the buildup of carbon dioxide in the atmosphere. Buying a fuel-efficient car—or better yet, a hybrid or electric one—not only reduces emissions but also conserves fuel and its associated costs. Replacing incandescent light bulbs with more energy-efficient fluorescent or LED bulbs will eliminate waste and conserve resources. And, of course, we should always recycle everything we can, including plastic, paper, cans, glassware, and electronics.

Given how important the environment is, it makes sense to attempt to understand it better; it makes even more sense to learn how to fix it. In an effort to do both, I recommend that everyone watch Al Gore's *An Inconvenient Truth* (2006), a documentary that discusses the environment and the effect that global warming is having upon it and, consequently, us as identified above.

If you want coverage of all aspects of the environment, read the news articles and blogs on the website for the Environmental Defense Fund (edf.org). If you're interested in wildlife conservation and how the environment affects it, visit the World Wildlife Fund (wwf.org).

I realize the preceding discussion is a lot of information to digest—try to take it in gradually. Once you have fully understood, accepted, and implemented my five principles, you'll broaden your knowledge of life and the world, thus helping you become a wiser person in the end. You'll also experience inner peace by drawing closer to God, thus sharing in His knowledge and love. This, in turn, will put you in closer touch with others and the environment, thus moving toward a state of oneness. Together, these accomplishments will give you the guidance necessary to make responsible choices in life and put you on the path toward spiritual enlightenment.

Chapter 7
Three Lessons

"One person can make a difference, and every person should try."

—John F. Kennedy

One important lesson humanity needs to better understand and more fully implement is sustainability. Whether it is drawing upon natural resources or expanding the size of a city, we must learn to do so in a way that can be supported over time. Uncontrolled growth is detrimental to everyone involved, even if the negative effects don't occur right away. We always have to think both short and long-term before planning something on a large scale. These factors are why I believe three very important spiritual lessons we need to learn from in this century are <u>global warming</u>, <u>overpopulation</u>, and <u>environmental degradation</u>. I refer to these lessons as spiritual because we will have to reach deep within our collective souls in order to solve them, much as we did during the civil rights movement of the 1950s and 60s. I have already discussed global warming in the previous chapter. As the name implies, it is affecting the planet on a global scale: glaciers are melting, seas are rising, weather is changing, and natural habitats are disappearing. What more evidence will it take? We will get a *lot* more than we bargained for if we do not do something significant about it well before this century is through.

Risk in Numbers

Overpopulation on a citywide scale has been around for centuries. Many cities simply build upward to accommodate the increase in people; others spread outward if they have the room to do so (known as "urban sprawl"). This leads to general overcrowding (e.g., of places such as stores and businesses) and congestion (e.g., of city streets), thus putting a strain on natural resources and resulting in an overall decrease in quality of life. There is no greater example of this than Europe in the 14th century. The world was subject to the onslaught of the Little Ice Age during that time, resulting in harsher winters and reduced harvests. Consequently, the Great Famine struck much of northwest Europe, and the productive capacity of the land and farmers wasn't sufficient to sustain the population. Because of a large population growth in the centuries leading up to that one and malnutrition due to famine, diseases such as the Black Plague quickly became epidemics, resulting in millions of deaths.

We see evidence of these events today, but on a much larger scale. Many developing countries are decimating their precious rain forests in an effort to procure land to accommodate urban sprawl and profitable farming. Disease control centers around the globe take comprehensive preemptive measures whenever the flu season strikes, in an urgent attempt to stave off potential pandemics. Problems like these are exacerbated by lots of people crowded into confined spaces. Why do you think farmers routinely feed their livestock antibiotics? Because they often get sick as a result of being cramped into tight living accommodations such that disease spreads easily from animal to animal. This over-medication leads, in turn, to more virulent strains of bacteria (i.e., 'superbugs') that are increasingly resistant to treatment. The Centers for Disease Control and Prevention report that at least 23,000 people die in the U.S. each year as a direct result of infection by such bacteria.

I believe there is only one reliable way to solve the overpopulation problem: family planning. Most people do not like to speak of such methods in this context, but it is the plain truth. Let me say here and now that I am not in favor of state-mandated population control measures; rather, I am talking about commonsense birth control methods. We as a people need to say "no" to arbitrarily large families. It is not up to me to decide what the recommended size should be, but it needs to be identified and followed if we are going to keep our population sustainable.

An organization leading the way toward supportable population growth is Population Connection. It is the largest grassroots population organization in the United States. Considering the global population surpassed 7,000,000,000 (i.e., *billion*) in 2011, and another million people are born into our world every 4.5 days (as of 2014), the primary goal of

Population Connection is "to stabilize world population at a level that can be sustained by Earth's resources." They work to ensure that every woman around the world who wants to limit her childbearing ability has access to the health services and contraceptive supplies she needs in order to do so. They find that typically, when women have access to affordable birth control, they have fewer children, regardless of income or educational levels. Some of their ongoing programs include increasing funding for both domestic and international family planning, creating comprehensive, progressive sex education programs, and convincing elected officials to sponsor legislation favoring family planning and population-related issues, to name a few. Their website is www.populationconnection.org.

Not surprisingly, a topic which immediately comes to mind when discussing overpopulation is environmental sustainability. Not only does overpopulation strain air, land, and water resources, it also pollutes them on a large scale. I have already discussed the buildup of carbon dioxide in the atmosphere and the resulting climate change. Industrial and farm runoff damages our streams, rivers, and lakes. Our environmental resources are not infinite, yet we treat them as such. We do not want to learn the lessons of sustainability passively; we want to respond to them proactively. If you've never witnessed a lush green meadow, a rich mountain lake, or a majestic waterfall, I highly recommend the experience. Becoming one with nature is among the most beautiful, peaceful experiences you can possibly imagine. God wants us to grow and prosper; we simply cannot do so over the long term unless we maintain the environment. The technology and know-how are already available; let's use them. Together, we can prevail over these challenges if we act now rather than later.

Chapter 8
Wants vs. Needs

"Try not to become a man of success, but rather a man of value."

—Albert Einstein

Frank P. Daversa

In the United States, we are fortunate to live in a free society. We enjoy freedom of speech, free and fair elections, and a free marketplace in which we can buy products or services we want and need. But along with freedom comes responsibility: we are responsible for thinking before we speak and act, for educating ourselves about the candidates and issues before we vote, and for choosing to spend our money wisely.

Unfortunately, too many of us can't quite manage that last responsibility. We are so inundated with advertisements and commercials everywhere we go that it's easy to want to buy whatever we can get our hands on. With the availability of credit and the Internet, we can purchase whatever we want whenever we want it, regardless of whether or not we can afford the purchases. It becomes all but impossible to distinguish between what we need to live our lives and what we want to make them more comfortable. Where do we draw the line between too much and too little?

The answer is <u>moderation</u>. We must focus first on what we *need* to purchase and then on the most worthwhile things we *want* to purchase—we don't need to have everything! That is called setting priorities. When we see an item on sale, it's easy to want to hoard it, but is this fair to other customers looking for the same thing? It's important to take time to reflect upon our actions so we can be sure we are making the right choices.

Greed Leads to Hedonism

One of the risks of a free-market society is hedonism. When we can get whatever we want, it becomes extremely easy for us to live our lives by the pleasure principle, focusing on short-term satisfaction rather than long-term needs. For example, some advertisers try to attract consumers by claiming their particular vacation offer or dessert is decadent; decadence neither develops a person's character nor strengthens his or her willpower. Hedonism goes hand in hand with materialism and greed, and focusing on material goods at the exclusion of more important aspects of life, such as faith, love, education, and financial responsibility, is truly self-defeating. Greed is often consistent with hoarding, and hoarding leads to excess and waste. These three aspects of life—hedonism, materialism, and greed—are signs of moral weakness, impairing the character and diminishing the spirit, resulting in a sense of complacency. Such behaviors reveal a lack of pride and result in a false sense of accomplishment.

Routinely buying items on a whim to satisfy our immediate gratification is a sign neither of moral excellence nor of personal growth. One such example is the preoccupation with "newness." A product is often deemed "better" just because it's new, or "obsolete" just because it's used or old. Such attitudes are perpetuated by advertisers who want you to buy their products *now.* There is probably no better example of this than fast food advertisements. Is having that double cheeseburger really necessary, or would a more heart-healthy meal suffice? And what happens to material goods once we replace them with new ones? They're too often discarded, a sign of how we've become a throwaway society. How much of what we routinely throw out could instead be recycled, reused, or donated to charity?

Don't Let Advertisers Tell You What to Think
A common advertising strategy is to lure consumers into making purchases based on their whims. Do you want to make life or financial decisions based on what unscrupulous advertisers tell you to think? Having the latest item on the market may be exciting, but is it truly necessary all the time? Products like computers become obsolete after about five years or so, therefore buying a new one in that time frame is understandable, but do you really need to spend money on the latest car or cell phone just because it's new, or will your current one do for a while longer?

Antique furniture is a good example of the value that older items possess. Do you know why an antique generally costs so much? Sure, it has to do with the principles of supply and demand, but what drives that demand? In a word:

character. Antiques possess a distinctive style and sense of history, qualities that are harder to find in more modern furniture. Just because a product is older does not mean it lacks value. Get the most out of your product's natural lifespan, and appreciate the intrinsic value it possesses beyond its material worth. That is not to say one should never purchase goods for pleasure; all it means is that such purchases should be made in moderation.

The best place to teach moderation is in our homes. The more we align our wants with our needs, the better the example we will set for our children. We buy goods on a regular basis, which provides the perfect opportunity for children to learn by example. Teach them to evaluate priorities. Life is all about balance: good vs. bad, a lot vs. a little, important vs. unimportant. The more balanced our lives are, the more we will be in harmony with the universe, and being in harmony with the universe is a big part of what spirituality is all about.

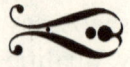

Chapter 9
The Relative Value of Success

"Keep in mind that neither success nor failure is ever final."

—Roger Babson

One thing many people say they want is success. But do we really need it to be happy? Success is a very tricky state because it is often fleeting. Take the media, for example: fads and trends come and go all the time, and unfortunately, so does fame. Rarely does success endure into old age for the few who are fortunate enough to achieve it. One big pitfall to success is that we have to spend a good portion of our time sustaining it. More often than not, this results in us making decisions that are contrary to our best interests. How many times has a "successful" person turned down a cherished pleasure or been unable to spend time with a loved one for the sake of a business meeting or a late night at the office? How many influential people have sold their souls to the Devil to get where they are?

Politicians who accept large campaign contributions from special interest groups to whom they then become beholden are a classic example of this. Another is the National Rifle Association (NRA), which has become completely beholden to gun manufacturers, to the point where the organization opposes commonsense gun reform measures like universal background checks on gun purchases. In the end, public entities such as these wind up serving their special interest lobbyists rather than the very constituents who helped bring them into power.

Success is often measured in terms of wealth, fame, and power. Lotteries are a quick and easy way to acquire riches, but they're hardly reliable—the chances of winning the jackpot are usually less than 1 in 100 million! Inheriting wealth is probably the easiest way to acquire riches, but of course you have to first be one of the fortunate few to be born into such a family. Becoming a movie star is another way, but a successful career in film is about as easy to achieve as winning the lottery; it takes many personal sacrifices and exceptional talent to make it to the top. Attaining power is a fourth way, but it often involves making lots of money, working your way to the top of a large organization, or achieving political success, none of which are easy to attain.

So how do people achieve success? Usually through hard work and dedication.

The Five Principles and Success

Let's use my five principles of spiritual enlightenment to assess the spiritual path of successful people. According to Answers.com, atheists and agnostics make up an estimated 14% of the world population, so extrapolating from there, it's safe to conclude that most people believe in God or at least in some greater power. Hence most successful people have incorporated principle #1: Accept God into your life and Jesus Christ as your savior.

According to the U.S. Census Bureau, the households and demographics with the highest educational achievement in the United States are also among those with the highest household income and wealth. Thus, while the population as a whole is proceeding further in formal educational programs, income and educational attainment remain highly correlated. The vast majority of the population, 85%, have finished high school. Contrast this with the 6% of the world population who have finished high school according to Answers.com. I expect this number to be higher in industrialized nations due to the greater incidence of wealth. Nevertheless, it appears that the presence of a high school education cannot always be assumed among the wealthy of the world. Most of the elite will have it, but some won't. Apparently, successful people do not consistently satisfy principle #2: Complete your formal education.

Many successful people seem to have it all: brains, beauty, and wealth. They have the finest education. They contribute to the betterment of society. They're loving parents to their children. However, other successful people seem to have difficulty conquering their personal demons. Some suffer from drug addiction. They are often burdened with scandal, as is evidenced by the fact that a substantial segment of the entertainment industry is devoted to covering just that. How many experience marital and/or family problems? One may argue that the general population does as well, but that is the point: such people are no better in this regard. While there are definitely successful people who are well developed intellectually, emotionally, and spiritually, some are no more enlightened than the rest of us with respect to principle #3: Learn more about yourself, your health and your mental well-being.

To their credit, many wealthy people give generously to charity and create or manage their own charitable foundations, but others are not as giving in critical ways. Many CEOs are against raising the minimum wage so that their hourly employees can live above the poverty line, which, in turn, would create more disposable income to help stimulate the economy. They object to universal health care, as beneficial as that would be for most, because it often involves a single-payer plan, which does not conform to the free-market model of economics. Wall Street bankers allowed their greed to manage their investments recklessly, which led to the 2008 Great Recession; millions of people suffered as a result. Such acts do not exhibit compassion toward our fellow human beings. Apparently principle #4, "Learn more about the needs of others," is not a prerequisite for becoming successful.

Many successful people support the environment wholeheartedly, but others definitely do not. There are those within commerce and industry who blatantly disregard the environment and see it as nothing more than an asset on a spreadsheet that they can exploit to their financial advantage. Big oil companies are a classic example of this. Chemical pollution and oil spills wreak havoc on the environment. Neither is principle #5, "Learn more about the natural environment in which we live," a prerequisite for becoming successful.

So as you can see, achieving enlightenment (as defined here) is not a requirement for success. Successful people do not consistently satisfy the five principles.

Many successful people are responsible, well-rounded individuals, and others are not. The good ones unfortunately suffer as a result of sins committed by the bad ones. The world has many deep-seated problems; we must all work together to solve them. The average person cannot tackle them alone; people in positions of authority need to lead the way in this regard. But we are not there yet. What, then, is the solution? Spiritual evolution. When humankind reaches the point where spiritual enlightenment is a prerequisite for achieving power, then the world will truly be a better place. In the meantime, concentrate on enlightening yourself and those you know.

Maybe someday in a later century this goal will be realized.

Success is not a true measure of inner peace and happiness. This is not to say we shouldn't pursue it if it comes our way—just keep the concept of success in perspective to other important attributes in life. We need to enjoy success while it lasts and refrain from defining ourselves in terms of it. We need to continue finding significance in simple pleasures, to strive for meaning in our lives, such as love, family, and friendships. We need to learn how to just *be*, living completely in the moment, perfectly content with who and where we are. This state is a challenge to attain in our hectic, 24/7 world.

Chapter 10
Love Relationships

"Being deeply loved by someone gives you strength, while loving someone deeply gives you courage."

—Lao Tzu

Relationships come in all types, depending on the context of the people involved.

By nature, most people are social creatures. We learn about relationships directly or indirectly from our environments, by trial and error as we grow up. Our family relations are generally the first we learn, and since we are almost entirely dependent as children on our surroundings for instruction, we are largely guided by our default spiritual paths.

Once we reach adolescence, we begin to exert a greater degree of independence as we exercise more free will. We have the chance to become liberated from our default paths, and therefore can begin changing our family relationships, sometimes for the better, sometimes for the worse. In many families, these years are marked by a good deal of turbulence as the child seeks to define his or her own identity. The combination of family counseling and spiritual enlightenment go a long way toward overcoming such obstacles.

Adolescence is also a time when we begin to take an interest in some of the most complicated relationships there are—romantic partnerships. Many of us learn how to interact with potential boyfriends or girlfriends by what we've learned in our home environment and/or by trial and error in the field. If the default example set in our homes was a constructive one, we have a good chance of learning how to relate positively with others; if it was bad, as was mine, we may have to wait until adulthood before we rise above our default paths and learn how to relate constructively.

My Struggle for Understanding
When I was a young man, I lacked a fundamental understanding of how to engage in a relationship with the opposite sex. It wasn't until I turned 25 that I met an older woman named Ollie who was willing to show me how to interact responsibly with a romantic partner. In essence, she helped me rise above my default spiritual path, and for that I will always be grateful. The benefit turned out to be mutual though, because she was more or less an A-type personality at the time and I showed her how to just *be*.

While I'd had a few close relationships up to that point, all less than a year in length, she and I quickly developed a unique psychological connection; it was then that I first found a prolonged state of oneness with a woman, an unparalleled experience. We were on the same page, the same wavelength, in complete harmony. Unfortunately, after 14 years, we grew apart, but we remain friends to this day. Regardless of what happened, I will never forget her or what we shared.

Years ago, dating used to largely be a hit-or-miss process. Now, with the advent of online dating services, that no longer needs to be the case. You can meet someone with a fair degree of certainty that you have found a reasonable match. The more effort you put into drafting a thoughtful dating profile and providing complimentary pictures of yourself on these websites, the more accurate your matches will be.

Keep in mind that all dating websites are *not* created equal; you may have to join more than one before finding a site that has the right members for you. Make sure you pick one that has a large selection of subscribers within your target age range and geographical area. Also, don't expect to meet Mr. or Mrs. Right on your first date—it may take a few months before you get the hang of it. The more you persevere, the better you chances will be. I have had success with dating sites, and you can, too.

The Five C's
Many factors go into making a good relationship—love, trust, dedication, sincerity and romance—as well as what I call the five C's:

1. **Compatibility**. In addition to having things in common, a good match must also have chemistry, a strong personal interaction, for the two people to relate well to one another.

2. **Communication**. A strong relationship must be based on communication, the ability to discuss the positive and negative aspects of the relationship in an open and constructive manner.
3. **Compassion**. Partners must share a sense of empathy with one another, an emotional bond toward the other person.
4. **Commitment**. Both partners must be dedicated to the success of the relationship so that it endures and will not flounder.
5. **Compromise**. The couple must be able to negotiate their differences fairly and amicably in order for the relationship to succeed.

These factors apply to platonic relationships as well as romantic ones. Romantically speaking, it's natural that no two people are the same, so at some point there are going to be differences. This is where good communication plays an important role. If you can't successfully resolve disputes, the relationship has a limited future, no matter how beneficial the good attributes of either partner. Communication contributes toward building understanding and trust between the two parties, which, combined with the other four C's, helps build a distinct and healthy affection that can last a lifetime.

Finding Lifelong Love

To ensure it will survive that long, the two partners need to commit to each other *only*. If the bond of love between two partners is strong, the relationship can lead to marriage, but if your prospective partner isn't able to follow the five C's, then he or she may not be ready for a serious relationship. One thing you *don't* want to do is rush into marriage. You'll have the rest of your lives to spend together; a year or so of preparation is not too much to ask.

The initial purpose of dating is to determine whether two people are sufficiently compatible with each other. With this in mind, if the two are young—say, 21 years old—it seems reasonable to date for at least six months and live together for another six months before getting married, which should provide sufficient time to really get to know one another and develop a sound understanding. You want to devote your marriage to growing together and sharing things in common, not uncovering major compatibility differences that should have been discussed beforehand. You'll also have the opportunity to save some much-needed money to begin your lives together.

Older couples—perhaps 40 years old—can probably shorten these times to five months each, because they generally have more experience in relationships and life. Since the number of singles over the age of 50 has grown with time, as evidenced by the rise of online senior dating services, more people in this age group are seeking relationships; they can probably shorten the above time frames a little further still because they possess even more experience. In any case, living together is a smart idea and serves as a good opportunity to determine whether a couple should get engaged. Couples should spend several more months affianced: It's a pivotal time to cement the bonds leading up to marriage, giving those involved the chance to prepare for their wedding ceremony/reception and discuss important beliefs such as whether and when the two want to start a family, their career goals and political affiliations.

Relationships and Spiritual Growth
Since relationships form such a big part of our lives, compatible couples should also focus on spiritual growth, which will help them form a deep and holistic bond. Ideally, you want to begin before you are engaged by following the first three principles of spiritual enlightenment: Accept God into your life and Jesus Christ as your savior; complete your formal education; and learn more about yourselves, your health and your mental well-being. Once you're married, you might, either on your own or as a couple, pursue the final two principles: Learn more about the needs of others, and learn more about the natural environment in which we live. If

you are still compatible after following the first three principles, then you will know you have a sound foundation upon which to build a lasting, satisfying relationship. You'll also be working toward becoming a strong match and attaining a state of oneness, a level of intimacy that can be difficult to achieve randomly on your own. Oneness can help two people grow closer and remain happy over time, thus improving their chances of a long, meaningful relationship that will last a lifetime. It's imperative that the two people see each other for who they really are, and decide if the person they see is someone they want to spend the rest of their lives with *before* getting married. As suggested above, this is a lot of ground to cover in the first pivotal year together—make the most of it.

Teach Your Children Well

One of the biggest responsibilities a couple can undertake is starting a family. While the early focus falls upon the child's immediate physical requirements, what about his or her psychological needs? Children need unconditional love and emotional support to bolster their delicate self-esteem. They need to know they will be loved whether their behavior is right or wrong.

Children are not born with instruction manuals, so common sense and knowledge of human behavior go a long way toward resolving their psychological needs. If you decide to have children, be prepared to show them lots of patience. They have much to learn, and they can only proceed at their own pace. Begin by acknowledging the fact that the younger the child, the more his or her needs come before yours.

Children require predictability in their lives. They need to know their next meal will be on the table, their favorite toy will be there to play with, and someone will be present to drop them off and pick them up from school when the time comes. This helps build confidence and trust.

Show an active interest in what happens in their lives. Ask them how their day went and what they did that was new. This demonstrates thoughtfulness and caring. Introduce the five principles of spiritual enlightenment to them. Start with the first one when they're young and advance to the remaining four as they get progressively older. This will provide a solid spiritual foundation on which to build. When they're old enough to understand, explain the reasons behind decisions you make. This shows them that there is a purpose to things and the world is not an arbitrary place.

Other supportive efforts include reading to the child to help build language comprehension, encouraging creative play to stimulate the child's imagination, and assigning light chores (like putting his or her toys away) to foster a sense of responsibility. Don't spoil or punish the child too heavily; once again, the key word here is *moderation*. The more rationally you behave toward your child, the more rational he or she will grow up to be. This thoughtful approach represents a place to start and will go a long way toward building character and a well-balanced child.

Chapter 11
Sins and Virtues, Religion and Death

"The best preparation for tomorrow is doing your best today."

—H. Jackson Brown, Jr.

Most of the spiritual concepts I know, I learned through hardship. Had I been fortunate enough to acquire spiritual knowledge sooner than I did, my default path might have been less arduous. Despite the effort involved, I am thankful for everything I have.

Regardless of your path, you should never take what you have for granted: Be grateful for your blessings, and approach life with a good degree of humility, which is an essential part of being spiritual. This trait consists of showing courtesy, modesty, and reverence toward others and toward moral principles such as faith, love, and compassion.

Real-life role models include Dr. Martin Luther King, Jr., Mahatma Gandhi, and His Holiness the Dalai Lama. All three devoted their lives to helping others in need. Bear in mind these individuals didn't learn humility overnight; it's a trait that takes time and patience to acquire.

Begin by appreciating the simpler pleasures in life, like a walk in the park, a child's joy, or a movie with a friend or loved one, and placing value in people and things that hold true meaning for you. Moreover, your expectations need to be realistic. Learn how to swallow your pride when the situation warrants. One of the many qualities my path taught me is humility. Understand it purposefully, not through adversity as I did. Do it right for all the reasons listed above, and it will become a way of life.

From Without or Within?

The battle between good and evil has existed since the dawn of humanity. But is this battle waged from within the individual or without? I contend that the battle between good and evil is primarily waged from within: Every person is born with the potential for good *and* evil. Barring genetic predispositions, these forces evolve within the person as he or she grows. Parenting and the environment in which people are raised play a vital role in determining which force wins out in the end.

The traditional tenets of Christian faith attribute at least some of these tendencies for sin to the influences of the Devil. I don't believe that God would allow a being who thrives on stealing souls on a grand scale, and leading people into temptation for all eternity, to co-exist within His kingdom. As with the principles of liberal Christian theology, I view the Devil metaphorically, as the potential for bad deeds in each of us.

I do, however, wholeheartedly believe in the existence of a place called Hell. Once we reach adulthood, each of us is the sole arbiter of whether we end up there or in Heaven. We need to take responsibility for our own actions. So the next time you pray for deliverance from the Devil, pray instead for the strength to overcome your own shortcomings and temptations for sin.

Frank P. Daversa

Seven Sins and Seven Virtues
If you've seen the movie *Se7en* (1995), you may already be familiar with the seven deadly sins: wrath, greed, envy, pride, lust, sloth and gluttony. These sins are not only examples of humanity's tendency to sin, but also, like the Ten Commandments, they serve as commonsense advice for living a strong, clean, spiritual life. In my belief system, those sins are distinctly human failings, not the Devil's handiwork. The Roman Catholic Church also recognizes the seven heavenly virtues, solutions for overcoming the seven sins:

— **Wrath** is inordinate and uncontrolled feelings of hatred, rage, and anger. According to the Catholic Church, you can correct this behavior by practicing the virtue of *patience*.
— **Greed** is a sin of excess: an extravagantly covetous desire for and pursuit of wealth, status, and power. Instead, practice *charity*.
— **Envy** is an insatiable desire for things that do not belong to you. People who commit this sin not only resent that another person has something they perceive themselves as lacking, but also wish the other person to be deprived of it. Instead, practice *kindness*.

- **Pride** means hubris, or exaggerated self-confidence, such as a desire to be more important or attractive than others, and a failure to acknowledge the good work of others. Instead, practice *humility*.
- **Lust** is the intense, generally sexual craving for someone or something and is characterized by vice. Instead, practice *chastity* (i.e., purity in conduct and intent; self-restraint).
- **Sloth** represents laziness and apathy, the failure to utilize one's talents and gifts. Instead, practice *diligence*.
- **Gluttony** is excessive eating or drinking, or the overconsumption of anything, concrete or intangible. Instead, practice *temperance*.

Needless to say, these negative behaviors are not in our best interests. At the minimum, practicing such evils would alienate us from people whose lives we affect; at the worst, they would place us on the path to Hell—at least in the eyes of the Catholic Church.

In truth, we all commit one or more of the seven deadly sins at some point in our lives; but if we commit them on a regular basis, it can be a sign of a more serious behavioral problem. If this sounds like you, you may want to consult a psychotherapist to increase your understanding of the causes behind these behaviors. A good therapist can help you uproot tendencies like the deadly sins and replace them with self-fulfilling personality traits, such as character and dignity and respect. The process starts by first recognizing these behaviors as self-defeating. We must then be willing to change for the better. We must practice the Golden Rule by treating others the way we would like to be treated ourselves. We all must work together effectively to achieve the common good. We all have the right to pursue a state of happiness, as long as we do so conscientiously and not at the expense of others.

The Goal of Religion
His Holiness the Dalai Lama offers perspective on religion. Many conflicts have been waged in the name of religion. Religions of the world, therefore, have a responsibility for behaving ethically. As the Dalai Lama said in *In My Own Words: An Introduction to My Teachings and Philosophy*,

> The purpose of religion is not to build beautiful churches and temples, but to cultivate positive human qualities such as tolerance, generosity, and love. Every world religion, no matter what its philosophical view, is founded first and foremost on the precept that we must reduce our selfishness and serve others. Unfortunately, sometimes

religion itself causes more quarrels than it solves. Practitioners of different faiths should realize that each religious tradition has immense intrinsic value and the means for providing mental and spiritual health.

One religion, like a single type of food, cannot satisfy everybody. According to their varying mental dispositions, some people benefit from one kind of teaching, others from another. Each faith has the ability to produce fine, warmhearted people; and despite their espousal of often-contradictory philosophies, all religions have succeeded in doing so. Thus, there is no reason to engage in divisive religious bigotry and intolerance, and every reason to cherish and respect all forms of spiritual practice.

Dogma aside, all religions have something valuable to contribute to humanity, such as faith in a greater power, compassion toward others, and assistance for the needy. The sooner they work together toward accomplishing these goals, the better it will be for us all.

Don't Fear the Reaper
Just as living is part of the cycle of life, so is death. It's an inescapable fact, yet few people think about it until their time draws near. It need

not be feared; whether we do depends on how well we prepared for it during our lifetimes. The more meaningful our lives, the less we will have to regret at the time of death. The way we feel when the time comes is very much dependent on the way we have lived. If we have sought enlightenment during our lives, we will be much more prepared for the afterlife. If, on the other hand, we have lived our lives by the pleasure principle, focusing primarily on sensory forms of input rather than core human values, we will naturally resist and even fear the end of the "pleasure cycle" when it finally comes.

As His Holiness the Dalai Lama explains in his book *In My Own Words: An Introduction to My Teachings and Philosophy*, your body is very precious to you. It has been your firmest, most reliable companion since conception. You have done much to give it the best care. You have fed it when it was hungry; you have given it drink when it was thirsty. You have rested when it was tired. You have been prepared to do anything and everything to attend to, comfort, and protect your body. In fairness, your body has also served you. It has almost always been ready to fulfill your needs. Just the function of the heart is a source of amazement. It's constantly at work, regardless of what you do, whether you're awake or asleep.

But when death strikes, our bodies give up. Our souls and our corporeal selves separate, and our precious vessels simply become useless corpses. In the face of death, your wealth and possessions, friends and relatives, and even your own body can do you no good. The only thing that can help us face the unknown is the faith we have developed in our hearts and the enlightenment we have cultivated in our souls. The two not only embolden our lives on Earth, but they also serve to guide us into the spiritual world. Spiritual growth enhances our minds and prepares us for what comes next.

Humans Attach Meaning

There is a concept in spirituality known as *attachment*. In practice, many people develop strong attachments to material things such as automobiles, clothes, and jewelry, among other tangible possessions. At the very least, that's because they cost a good deal of money. Unfortunately, this behavior tends to lead to the principle of "more is never enough." In so doing, we place control in external belongings instead of within ourselves. Let me be clear: there is nothing wrong with having material possessions; we just shouldn't define ourselves in terms of them. Draw the line between wanting something and needing it for some form of social approval.

We also feel attachment toward the intangible: nationality, culture, religion, etc. People take such identities seriously, as well they should. But consider how many wars have been fought over one or more of these issues. We must never lose sight of the fact that there is one thing that everyone has in common: We are all human beings before we are Americans, Russians, Chinese, Catholics, Arabs, Jews, etc. We can value these traits as long as we don't define our totality in terms of them. Allow your compassion for your fellow humans to reach beyond national or religious labels and realize our underlying humanity. There would be far fewer conflicts in the world if people would only adopt this point of view!

Forgiveness and Compassion
There is truth behind the adage, "To err is human, to forgive is divine." Forgiveness demonstrates a sense of compassion for those with whom we share this planet. Its benefits are twofold: When you forgive, you relinquish blame toward another party who may have done you or others harm. This opens the door to a much more positive interaction with them, should you so desire. Second, you let go of negative thoughts and feelings you're harboring toward that individual or group. Maintaining such negative "vibes" can only cause you emotional harm. Forgiveness is a clear exercise in the Golden Rule (see below) and a sense of moral responsibility.

His Holiness the Dalai Lama provides some perspective on the subject in *Beyond Religion: Ethics for a Whole World:*

> When you dwell on the harm someone has done to you, there is an inevitable tendency to become angry and resentful at the thought. Yet clinging to painful memories and harboring ill will [does] nothing to rectify the wrong committed and will have no positive effect on you. Your peace of mind will be destroyed, your sleep will be disturbed, and eventually even your physical health is likely to suffer. If, on the other hand, you are able to overcome your feelings of hostility toward wrongdoers and forgive them, there is an immediate and perceptible benefit to you. By leaving past actions in the past and restoring your concern for the well-being of those who have done you wrong, you gain a tremendous feeling of inner confidence and freedom, which allows you to move on as your negative thoughts and emotions tend to dissipate.
>
> Remember, forgiveness does not mean we condone what was done, only that we have come to terms with the fact that the responsible parties behaved in the only way they understood how at the time, as unpleasant as that might have been. It's important that we do forgive freely and move on with our lives, without holding grudges. The

same principles apply with respect to forgiving ourselves; it's important to relinquish feelings of self-condemnation. Life is best lived with a clear mind and conscience.

The Meaning of the Golden Rule

"Do unto others as you would have them do unto you." The Golden Rule shouldn't be taken as an imposition of our will upon others; its purpose is to help us be more conscientious and capable of thinking of the best interests of others as well as our own. Just as importantly, following the Golden Rule demonstrates a level of spiritual development on our part. Simply put, do it because it's the right thing to do.

One way to convey thoughtfulness for others is by performing simple acts of kindness, such as holding the door open for someone or allowing a car to turn in front of you on a busy street. Friendliness is an expression of generosity and divine love. Making someone's day by being courteous is good for our souls. Don't hesitate to say "please," "thank you," "excuse me," and "you're welcome" on a regular basis. These basic pleasantries really help to make the world a better place.

Music and Spirituality

Music has been a vital part of my life. In my difficult youth, it was one of the few things that kept me centered. The right kind of music can be very influential in putting us into a spiritual state of mind. Try selections that are inspirational, yet soothing. I find New Age and classical music to be helpful in this regard. Music is more accessible than at any other point in history. With the development of portable media players, we can listen to music almost anywhere, so take advantage of it.

Politics and Spirituality

There are several constants in life—death, taxes, the ever-changing seasons—and then there is change itself. It can happen slowly, such as geologic erosion, or quickly, such as the half-life of a heavy element. It can be positive, lateral, or negative. It is a fact of life everyone must embrace, yet there are those who refuse to accept it. For example, a significant number of people appear to resist the changing demographics in America. Whites are slowly but surely becoming a minority, especially in big cities. That is why those who oppose this trend often support onerous voter ID laws. As drafted, voter ID laws and general voter suppression tactics specifically disenfranchise Blacks as well as other minorities, the young, and the elderly in ways not seen since the original Voting Rights Act of 1965 was passed. This is clearly a step backward for these people, not forward. It does not demonstrate compassion toward your fellow human beings, it is not the kind of equality Dr. Martin Luther King, Jr. fought for, nor is it consistent with spiritual principles. Another reason disenfranchised voters are being cast aside is that they are typically not big campaign donors and thus do not have a lot of political influence. Those responsible for these infringements on society let their thirst for electoral (and hence political) power deny civic-minded citizens their constitutional rights. Voting is a right, not a privilege, and should be treated as such.

Then there is lateral change (i.e., change for change's sake). I would argue that many new hairstyles fall into this category. If they were genuinely better than those that preceded them, people would wear them indefinitely. How many times have you witnessed old photographs and remarked how funny the subject's hair looks? In contrast, some hairstyles seem to stand the test of time and can be worn at almost any stage in history.

The most revered change is positive. The Emancipation Proclamation and the Civil Rights Act of 1964 are classic examples. One civil rights issue I would argue falls in this category is LGBTQ+ rights and same-sex marriage. Before you can effectively address this issue, however, one fact must be made clear: Homosexuality is not a lifestyle choice; it is involuntary. A gay person cannot become straight any more than the Earth can stop orbiting the sun. Homosexuality is a fact of life and will continue to exist as long as people do. We must stop treating LGBTQ+ individuals as half-citizens; as members of society, they deserve the same rights afforded everyone else. If you embrace your spirituality, you will overcome the obstacles presented by change and likewise embrace the LGBTQ+ community's crusade for equality.

Government is the lifeblood of any nation, and politics are at the heart of any government. America's two-party system has been in place since 1854. Each party believes it knows what is right for the nation. Since they largely disagree as to what that might be, the two parties have been at each other's throats for much of the time since then. Which one is right? The answer to that question lies with the individual voter based on a thorough understanding of the issues and candidates involved. But one thing is certain: if the country (and hence the society) is to grow and prosper, the two parties must cooperate. As much as the United States has evolved since its inception, we still face many problems. We depend on our elected officials to address these problems and come up with effective solutions. That is why the people we elect to office are so important. But no single party can solve these problems alone; it takes at least two to tango. Cooperation and compromise are imperative if the government is to function effectively. The most productive solutions are those that address the common good. When political parties cater to special interests in contrast to the majority's needs, the system usually fails to uphold that good. If we are to grow as a nation economically, socially, and spiritually, we must all work together to benefit the well-being of our citizens. We must overcome the constraints of fear. We must put aside partisanship and confront the issues facing us so that we may propel this country to even greater heights. We need to all get along.

I have identified a pattern of change involving politics. It concerns the development of public freedoms. I believe God allows a particular party to come into power when He wants to grant certain rights to us. When we reach a point at which we begin taking these rights for granted, He allows the other party to come into power to effectively take them away, until such time as we are willing to fight for them again. Low voter turnout is a classic example of this. The right to vote is fundamental to our democracy. Voter apathy severely diminishes that right. That's why key provisions of the 1965 Voting Rights Act were struck down by the Supreme Court in 2013. The law will remain that way until such time as we fully respect the right to vote again. As long as we behave this way, there will always be a viable opposition party. This is part of the cycle of life. That's why history often repeats itself: it is God's way of teaching us the lesson over and over again, until we get it right. It's all part of God's plan. So what is the moral to this story? Treasure your freedoms, or else you run the risk of losing them.

Three issues are at the forefront of the political debate. The importance of education, the environment, and assistance for the poor cannot be overemphasized. Unfortunately, there are elected officials who try to politicize these issues by seriously cutting back essential funding for each. Beware of such officials; they place their rigid ideology ahead of the common good. In other words, do not support any fiscal policy or politician who does not support these three issues wholeheartedly. They are a vital part of our spiritual future and deserve our full backing.

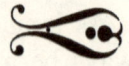

Chapter 12
Truth and Growth

"We are not human beings having a spiritual experience; we are spiritual beings having a human experience."

—Teilhard de Chardin

Modern life barrages us with an abundance of information, much of the time in excess. Sometimes there seems to be more than one truth to it all—how can we sort through it and tell what is truthful and what is not? Common sense and wisdom go a long way toward that goal. Despite what we may be led to think, I believe there exists an absolute truth to all life, and only God knows it. The further we grow spiritually, the more we begin to comprehend that truth.

We Must Seek Our Own Truths
Some people claim to know the truth when in reality what they say is subjective. I have always been a seeker of truth—not just conventional wisdom, but objective truth. I have tried to include as much of it as possible within this book. To acquire truth for ourselves, we first have to know how to seek out knowledge. To begin with, we mustn't be afraid to ask questions. Our source should be willing to offer information readily; beware of sages who answer in riddles—they're just dodging the question.

One way to improve our thinking skills is to broaden our understanding and experiences. It's easier to determine whether information is true if we have facts in our heads to which we can compare it. The more knowledgeable we are, the better judgment we can exercise.

Frank P. Daversa

We should also not be afraid of questioning the status quo. When it comes to religious institutions, many principles are passed down from one generation to the next without question. Do these religious doctrines represent truth or merely long-accepted dogma? For instance, is it really a sin, as the Catholic Church contends, for a couple to live together before marriage? What better way to determine whether they are truly compatible with each other so they can enter into a long and lasting state of holy matrimony? More questions arise about church doctrine regarding the role of women and such topics as sex, birth control, gay rights, and evolution, just to name a few.

This is not to say that organized religion is disadvantageous to our lives; we need to choose which doctrines within our faith are reasonable and just—in other words, which ones represent truth for all. If you don't follow a particular faith, then you need to choose which long-standing spiritual practices hold true for you.

The Path to Truth

There are those who say that since there are many spiritual paths to follow, no objective truth or absolute exists to determine which is better. On the contrary, I strongly believe there exists a better path: the one which leads you most directly to a state of spiritual enlightenment. Understand that you'll encounter many ups and downs along the way. One of my objectives in writing this book is to maximize your highs and minimize your lows, to make spirituality as rewarding for you as it is for me. Remember, the primary goal here is to achieve truth and understanding. I believe growth leads a person to truth, and spiritual enlightenment is growth, therefore spiritual enlightenment results in truth.

We may ask ourselves what is the point of growing spiritually if we don't need our spirituality until we die. The answer is: Because our souls live within us from the moment we're born. Our minds grow intellectually, our bodies grow physically, and our souls grow spiritually. In addition to personal spiritual growth, we can grow spiritually in our societal and global dealings. Societal growth consists of citizens working together to understand social issues and solve problems, such as crime, drugs, poverty, illiteracy, and discrimination. Global growth consists of citizens from all nations uniting and working together to understand international issues and solve problems that plague the world, such as war, human rights abuses, global warming, poverty, and hunger. Only when we begin to solve these problems together will we truly evolve as a people and as a species.

Signals from God
Some people such as atheists question the very existence of God. They contend if He is real, He would show Himself to us. They keep searching for a sign. In fact, the signs are all around us. Every major human success or disaster represents such a sign; all we need to do is heed them. God pays close attention to how we respond to these events when they occur.

It's not up to us to determine how God should and should not behave; He is the Supreme Being, and He decides what He needs to do at any given point in time. Consider what would happen if God did elect to present Himself to us. There are so many entrenched, seemingly insurmountable problems in this world that we would immediately run to Him for help. We would become completely dependent upon His infinite resources to cure humanity's ills. For that matter, this is essentially the same reason we have not, to my knowledge, been contacted (at least in recent history) by other intelligent life forms in the universe. God will not allow that to happen until we more or less get our acts together here at home.

God wants us to be self-sufficient. He wants us to be able to solve our problems on our own. We did so in WWII against global imperialism, we did so during the Cuban missile crisis against the threat of nuclear war, we did so following 9/11 against the war on terror, and we can do so again.

The human spirit is resourceful and indomitable. The very act of responsibly conquering our problems will make it possible for God to formally show Himself to us when He deems the time is right. In the meanwhile, let's concentrate on doing what needs to be done in the present, planning for the future, and preparing for the afterlife.

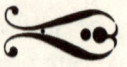

Chapter 13
Intolerance

*"The highest result of
education is tolerance."*

—Helen Keller

Spirituality in the 21st Century

Of all the problems that exist in the world today, there is one so pervasive that it touches almost everyone in one way or another. It has been around since the dawn of humanity. Wars have been fought because of it. It's handed down from generation to generation. It manifests itself on both an individual and a societal level. This problem is *intolerance*.

Intolerance is the unyielding adherence to one's opinions or prejudices, regardless of how damaging they might be. Its development can be summed up by the age-old expression, "Which came first, the chicken or the egg?" Intolerance is often passed down from parent to child. If one or both parents are intolerant, then they won't be accepting of a variety of behaviors in their children. This, in turn, hurts and frustrates the child, and over a sufficient period of time may cause him or her to either become intolerant like his or her parents or subservient, giving in to his or her parents' demands. If the child does not become adequately aware of his or her own behaviors, he or she can grow up to repeat the cycle.

Tolerance, on the other hand, is the act of acceptance—the measure of a person's ability to effectively deal with difficulty. Raising children can be very demanding; they require much love and lots of patience so they can develop properly. Take away patience, and the individual is frequently left with intolerance; without patience, the vicious cycle begins. In order to effectively teach our children tolerance and stop the cycle, we have to be willing to practice it ourselves. This means challenging our beliefs about self-defeating attitudes and behaviors. If left unchecked, intolerance can lead to hatred, prejudice, religious persecution, discrimination, sexism and homophobia.

Peace, Love, and Understanding

An important part of spirituality is being at peace with ourselves and the world, not exercising hostility toward either. Lasting tranquility is not possible without first achieving inner peace. For example, it is not possible to achieve this goal if we are filled with hostility.

Although peacefulness and tolerance go hand in hand, unfortunately so do animosity and intolerance. Animosity constitutes an antagonistic or hostile attitude toward another person or thing. It is not consistent with acceptance or tolerance.

If enough people develop intolerant behavior, they can band together to form hate groups. If even more become intolerant, then such behavior can escalate to a societal scale, resulting in things such as slavery, Jim Crow laws, the Ku Klux Klan, neo-Nazi groups, and white supremacist groups. I turn to His Holiness the

Dalai Lama for a perspective on anger. In *Beyond Religion: Ethics for a Whole World,* he says:

> What anger most depends on for its perpetuation is our own inner dissatisfaction, [a] state of latent irritation or lack of contentment . . . It is this general underlying mental unease which makes us susceptible to the triggering of destructive emotions, especially anger. Such inner dissatisfaction is the fuel upon which destructive emotions such as anger and hostility depend. Therefore, just as extinguishing the initial sparks is a more effective method of preventing fire damage than waiting until the fire is blazing, in the same manner; dealing with the underlying causes of discontent is a more effective way to prevent destructive emotions from doing damage than waiting until the emotions become full blown.

In other words, an ounce of prevention is worth a pound of cure. In order to eradicate destructive emotions, challenge the beliefs which lead to such feelings before they happen and replace them with more constructive beliefs, thus increasing your self-awareness in the process.

Frank P. Daversa

Awareness Is the Answer
Self-awareness is crucial for preventing and eliminating intolerance. We can't solve a problem until we know it exists. Ignorance fuels intolerance. It can inhibit our sense of awareness and stunt our growth—if we're unreceptive when faced with new information, we won't become aware and grow.

Knowledge is essential to wisdom, and wisdom is essential to spirituality. Spirituality is all about being in touch with the world around you. Connect with your environment and the broader community of humankind. Since tolerance is a vital part of compassion for others, and compassion is a vital part of spirituality, tolerance is vital to spirituality. Together, these concepts are at the heart of my second, third, and fourth principles of spiritual enlightenment.

An organization instrumental in spreading awareness of tolerance is the Southern Poverty Law Center, accessible at www.splcenter.org. It's a nonprofit organization founded in 1971 to ensure that the promises of the civil rights movement in this country become a reality for all. Its members are dedicated to fighting hate and bigotry, and to seeking justice for the most vulnerable members of society. Their renowned tolerance program teaches tolerance, reduces prejudice, improves intergroup relations, and fosters school environments that are inclusive and nurturing for our nation's children. They have an extensive news library located on their website under the "What We Do" and "Our Issues" sections.

The question is, do we want to live life full of happiness or hostility? Our society is still filled with intolerance against minorities, LGBTQ+ individuals, illegal immigrants, and others. For example, Blacks have been disenfranchised and underprivileged throughout history, including the present. They are often unfairly targeted by law enforcement. Are we going to merely accept such practices or challenge them and become better citizens as a result? There is no room for complacency in this regard. We cannot rest on our laurels and take for granted accomplishments made by previous generations. We conquered many forms of prejudice following the Civil War and the civil rights movement, but our work is not done. Ultimately, we need to ask ourselves, "Does there need to be more or less tolerance in God's universe?" The only rational and humane answer to that question is "more."

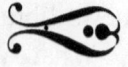

Chapter 14
Levels and Learning

"The ultimate measure of a man is not where he stands in moments of comfort and convenience, but where he stands at times of challenge and controversy."

—Martin Luther King, Jr.

God designed the world with obstacles so that we would learn from them and grow. As the French philosopher Pierre Teilhard de Chardin once said, "We are not human beings having a spiritual experience. We are spiritual beings having a human experience." Earth is merely a learning ground for humanity, so that we can evolve spiritually before moving on to the afterlife. I trust this is part of God's plan. Just as there are many grades or levels of education, there are many levels of spiritual development.

Death does not mean the end of our souls' learning and growing. Depending upon the level we were at in life at the time we passed away, there is a spiritual level in the afterlife for everyone—that's another reason why we should grow as much as we can while we're here. That way, we can progress to a higher level in the afterlife, along with leaving behind a positive footprint on Earth.

Whether it happens quickly or it takes a longer time, God will see to it that each of us grows. Once we've achieved a certain degree of growth in the afterlife, our soul advances to the next level. We continue moving on to higher levels as we evolve spiritually. If we don't progress, we remain at the same level until we grow as God intended—this is where you would typically be reincarnated if He so chooses. Many levels exist here on Earth, but there are an infinite number in the afterlife, with God's being the highest.

Passive vs. Proactive Learning

As is the case with any form of education, learning involves lessons. We often learn from the choices we make. For instance, do we hire a qualified job applicant who happens to be Black or LGBTQ+, or do we go with a lesser-qualified white, straight applicant instead? Do we stop to call 911 for a person involved in an auto accident or do we just keep driving? Do we set aside money to give to charity or do we spend it on something trivial? In particular, we can either take an active approach toward learning our spiritual lessons or we can leave it up to fate to guide us; in other words, we can learn them *proactively* or *passively*. Clearly, it would appear the proactive approach is God's preferred method of learning. As indicated above, I believe God has defined certain lessons He wants us to learn at different times along the way. Each lesson corresponds to the personal, societal, or global domains mentioned previously. If we learn the lesson correctly, we move on to the next one. If we do not, we will be obligated to continue trying until we get it right. Either way, God will ensure that the lesson will be learned.

There is no better example of this than global warming, as already mentioned. I firmly believe, if left unabated, that persistent inaction on our part will lead not only to severe environmental consequences, but also a mass extinction of life on Earth. The harm done to the environment will create violent weather patterns which, in turn, will cost many lives. Probably the worst consequence of this change in weather will be widespread crop failures that will result in food shortages, which will leave millions of people without an adequate supply of food. Habitats will become barren. Seas will rise, resulting in extensive flooding. Wildfires will proliferate. Put bluntly, all Hell will break loose. Much of this will take place in the second half of the century, although the warning signs are there already. We have between now and then to get off our collective asses and conscientiously *do* something about it. I cannot emphasize this enough. We do not want to incite the wrath of God. He has an agenda He wants us to follow. We must either adhere to that agenda, or suffer the consequences. If we take the necessary steps to avert these dangers, He will work with us to devise solutions to the problem. He wants to help, but we must first demonstrate the willingness to *try* and save the planet. It will take a concerted global effort to find such solutions. The 2016 Paris climate accord was an important first step. We conquered a global threat once before during WWII, and we can do it again.

The resulting food shortage underscores two outstanding problems: climate change (as stated) and overpopulation. God allowed us to get into a situation in which global warming would develop so that we may learn from it once and for all. If we respond proactively, then the problem will be averted and we would get to lead normal, happy lives. If, on the other hand, we respond passively, the problem will escalate and we will be forced to do something about it after it has gotten way out of hand, resulting in a grand loss of life. Such a loss would be of no great consequence to the Lord because some of these people would simply go to heaven and the rest would be reincarnated. While God views all life as sacred, He would see it as a necessary sacrifice for the sake of saving the planet, a prime directive. If this warning sounds intimidating, then it should be. The well-being of the Earth is at stake. It is imperative we practice the concept of sustainability. So what, then, is to be learned from all this? Conserve the damn planet, and conserve it *now*.

World Wars
As alluded to above, when we learn passively, we rely on our default paths, and we will then be destined either to repeat the lesson or learn it the hard way. Many wars fall into this category. How many did not solve the problem that initially created them, or resulted in even more problems after the fact? Others ended up solving problems, but at what cost? I believe World Wars I and II were two large-scale lessons in the 20th century that God wanted us to learn from once and for all. There were many big, long-standing evils in the world at that time that needed to be corrected. Humanity lacked sufficient insight to resolve these inherent flaws without first resorting to conflict. Central and Axis powers were driven by deep-seated aggression and hatred rather

Spirituality in the 21st Century

than peace. Tensions in Europe ran high, war was inevitable in both cases. Volumes have been written about the pros and cons of each war. But if I had to summarize in three words the shortcomings that led to both, they would be tyranny, appeasement, and imperialism. Tyranny and imperialism almost always result in a violation of fundamental human rights.

These forms of aggression have plagued humanity for millennia. Such aggression has failed time and time again throughout history, even if it took decades or centuries to overcome. In my opinion, growing this way represents a low level of spiritual development, and is a case for learning passively. It is obvious that world powers did not adequately learn their lessons from WWI, since WWII began less than 21 years later. Had humankind been motivated by its spirituality instead of its ego, the outcome of both wars might have been much better, if not averted altogether. Despite the fact that the two wars were won by the Allies, world powers did not fully heed the aforementioned threats in advance, so many nations had to pay a heavy price to defeat these threats after the fact. That is not to say that such perils do not still exist today, but at least they do not take place on a global scale.

On the other hand, if we learn proactively, we will rise above our default spiritual paths and we will get the chance to lead happy, fulfilling lives. In order to solve the global problems God has laid out for us, we must work together as a people. An example of learning proactively and working together is the 1991 Persian Gulf War. The global community mobilized its forces against a tyrant before it was too late, and the result was a war that lasted only a few months with minimal casualties. Furthermore, because it was done correctly the first time, the problem remained solved (the 2003 Iraq war notwithstanding). If humankind could only have approached all wars this way, think of how many could have been prevented or at least minimized, and the suffering and costs that would have been avoided.

The question remains, why does God let events like these happen in the first place? It's well within His power to prevent them. The simple answer: He wants us to learn from them. We live in a violent world. Violence inundates our everyday lives, from news to video games to television to movies. We have not reached the level of development at which we respond exclusively to nonviolent messages.

Take the three major stock market crashes of 1929, 1987, and 2008. Financial prognosticators warned of imminent doom before each crash, and yet did we sufficiently heed their advice? No. Simply put, adversity and violence are the lessons we seem to learn from most. Until we consistently demonstrate otherwise, we will continue to learn by such measures.

Following the 1999 Columbine High School massacre, school security was tightened, but was it enough? No. The 2007 Virginia Tech massacre happened eight years later; were the security measures taken following that shooting sufficient? No. The 2012 Sandy Hook Elementary School massacre happened five years after that. Were the preventive measures taken in response to that shooting enough? No, as was evidenced by the 2016 Pulse nightclub massacre. It's a complex problem that requires a comprehensive solution. To start with, the mental condition of the shooter needs to be addressed and understood well. Also, states need to provide ample funding for mental health services. Background checks need to be performed on every gun purchase. Such measures will not infringe upon the public's second amendment rights in any way. One fact is clear: the United States has far more guns than any other industrialized nation. With all these guns circulating, something bad is bound to happen. Does the average citizen need military-style semi-automatic assault rifles with high-capacity magazine clips? Certainly not. While an assault weapons ban might not prevent all massacres like these from happening again, such an effort is a good, commonsense approach. If implemented, we must resolve to enforce the ban over the long run and not allow it to expire like the 1994 law simply because of a change in administration.

The latest massacre is not the first time this has happened, and it won't be the last until we as a society solve this problem for good.

Sometimes the lessons we are presented with take place on a grand scale (wars are a classic example, as previously stated). One event of this kind was the September 11, 2001 World Trade Center terrorist attacks. You may ask, why did God let that happen? Because terrorist organizations such as al-Qaeda had been on the rise for many years and the tragedy focused the world's attention on the dangers of terrorism like a laser beam. Something had to be done to stop these organizations from evolving into a global threat. Imagine the untold carnage if one of them got their hands on a nuclear weapon and used it. Hundreds of thousands, if not millions, of people could be killed as a result. Comprehensive measures have been taken to prevent such attacks although, as we know, they still happen. As a result, terrorism continues to be a constant threat and we must remain ever vigilant. One problem that has not been adequately addressed is the vast difference in wealth between privileged and underprivileged countries of the world. As discussed in principle #4—"Learn more about the needs of others"—problems will always exist so long as there is a large divide between the haves and have-nots. Simply put, desperate people tend to take desperate measures to advance their cause.

Death Is Just the Beginning

Our ultimate goal should be to live long, healthy, prosperous lives, and it's a real tragedy when so many lives are cut short like those mentioned. Untimely death is often hard to accept, but there is no need to mourn for very long. We should be consoled by the strong likelihood that the victims of tragedy are in a better place afterwards, and the day may come when we will get to join them. I firmly believe that lives given in the service of the Lord are rewarded a place in Heaven. The abrupt termination of life on Earth is an understandable price to pay for eternal life in complete paradise at God's side.

Keep in mind that we have to be chosen by God to receive such a fate; we can't cause it to happen artificially, such as by committing suicide, an act that is expressly forbidden. God gave us life; it's his to take back when He sees fit. Suicide unnaturally cuts short God's lessons for us on Earth, which means we'll serve penance in Hell or be reincarnated onto a less favorable spiritual path—or both.

No matter how bad your current path may be, it's not worth taking your own life. You can't predict what life has in store for you; better things may come your way down the road. Never give up hope. There *are* solutions to your problems—you just have to find them. Seek help—don't attempt to tackle them all on your own. If you feel this way, try consulting with a trained therapist or life counselor. They can help you find a good reason for living. Before you consider taking your own life, think of the enormous, adverse impact your death will have on the loved ones you leave behind. It's easy to feel hopeless; just remember, God believes in you. If you should need immediate assistance, call the National Suicide Prevention Hotline in the U.S. anytime at 1-800-273-TALK (8255). Do you want to risk forfeiting your life for naught? You must keep reminding yourself of the concept of eternity. Is ending your unfortunate path in life worth forsaking eternity in Heaven next to God?

There are no shortcuts to Heaven. The best way to get there is to overcome your obstacles, learn your lessons well, and grow spiritually. Follow the many principles outlined in this book and you will be on your way toward a productive life on Earth and a more favorable place in the afterlife.

Chapter 15
Conclusion

"To accomplish great things, we must not only act, but also dream; not only plan, but also believe."

—Anatole France

Our bodies exist on Earth for a short time compared to how long our souls live in the afterlife, so we must make the most of our time while we are here. Our souls' potential is boundless; God designed them that way. To make our terrestrial journeys meaningful, everyone should have the opportunity to live life to its fullest. What better way to live than to grow as a person and be all you can be? It is best to develop holistically, not just in one direction or two. Become well-rounded. Develop a curiosity toward life and how it works. It may be customary to grow mentally and physically, but what about spiritually? We need to develop our minds and bodies for life on Earth, and develop our souls for our time here and thereafter. Doing so places us closer to God, making it possible to share in His knowledge of the world and even the universe. After all, are these pursuits not the ultimate goal?

If you have followed the many principles presented in this book closely, you now see it's possible to understand spirituality and life in a meaningful way. You understand the implications of your default spiritual path on the rest of your life. You have a strong belief in God and Jesus. You will pursue your formal education if you have not done so already. You better understand your mind and what makes it behave the way it does. You have a greater compassion toward others, and appreciation for the environment. You understand three spiritual lessons Earth needs to address in the 21st century. You are able to better balance your needs vs. your desires. You have a better understanding of love relationships. You better understand how to deal with the prevalence of intolerance in our world. You are able to distinguish between passive and proactive learning and better interpret God's messages for us as a result. In short, you have undoubtedly grown personally and spiritually.

This book is designed to make you think honestly about your life and the role spirituality plays in it. Wisdom leads to empowerment, and empowerment leads to enlightenment. Empowering yourself is one of the most enriching and liberating experiences you can possibly undertake. Since the path to spiritual enlightenment often has many twists and turns, it is my greatest wish that this book empowers you to accomplish this noble effort in as rewarding and straightforward a manner as possible. The concepts presented herein are not tentative; they are meant to be implemented throughout your lifetime. Embrace them gradually but diligently, and become a better individual because of it. Never give up; *persevere* always. As you progress down your path, bear in mind that the ideas contained within do not constitute the end of your spiritual journey, but rather just the beginning . . .

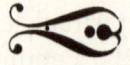

Recommended Reading

Throughout the manuscript, I've mentioned several texts, and have paraphrased from others, that I have found to be excellent reading:

A Guide to Rational Living, by Albert Ellis, Ph.D., and Robert A. Harper, Ph.D. (Wilshire Book Co., 1997).

Ansel Adams: 400 Photographs, by Ansel Adams, edited by Andrea G. Stillman (Little, Brown and Company, 2007).

Beyond Religion: Ethics for a Whole World, 1st Edition, His Holiness the Dalai Lama (Houghton Mifflin Harcourt, 2011).

Dating, Mating, and Relating: How to Build a Healthy Relationship, by Albert Ellis, Ph.D., and Robert A. Harper, Ph.D. (Citadel, 2003).

How to Practice: The Way to a Meaningful Life, 1st Edition, His Holiness the Dalai Lama (Atria Books, 2002).

In My Own Words: An Introduction to My Teachings and Philosophy, 3rd Edition, His Holiness the Dalai Lama (Hay House, Inc., 2008).

www.ingramcontent.com/pod-product-compliance
Lightning Source LLC
Chambersburg PA
CBHW030119100526
44591CB00009B/455